The Molecular Biology of the Major
Histocompatibility Complex of Domestic Animal Species

The Molecular Biology of the Major Histocompatibility Complex of Domestic Animal Species

Edited by **CAROL M. WARNER**
MAX F. ROTHSCHILD
SUSAN J. LAMONT

 Iowa State University Press / Ames

Carol M. Warner is professor of biochemistry at Iowa State University.
Max F. Rothschild is professor of animal science at Iowa State University.
Susan J. Lamont is associate professor of animal science at Iowa State University.

This text was provided in camera-ready form by the authors.

The papers in this volume were presented at a symposium held at Iowa State University, Ames, Iowa, on October 23–24, 1987.

First edition, 1988

Library of Congress Cataloging-in-Publication Data

The molecular biology of the major histocompatibility complex of domestic animal species / edited by Carol M. Warner, Max F. Rothschild, Susan J. Lamont — 1st ed.
     p. cm.
    "Papers in this volume were presented at a symposium held at Iowa State University, Ames, Iowa, on October 23–24, 1987" — T.p. verso.
    ISBN 0-8138-0304-7
    1. Major histocompatibility complex — Congresses. 2. Veterinary immunogenetics — Congresses. 3. Molecular genetics — Congresses. I. Warner, Carol M., 1946– . II. Rothschild, Max Frederick, 1952– . III. Lamont, Susan J., 1953– .
SF757.234.M64 1988   88–26589
636.089′6079 — dc19   CIP

CONTENTS

v

PART 2□ ABSTRACTS

Photographs from the conference appear at the end of Part 1.

PREFACE

The major histocompatibility complex (MHC), first discovered in mice just over 50 years ago, is one of the most important sets of genes involved in the genetic control of the immune response. Elucidation of the structure and function of the genes and protein products of the MHC has been a major goal of immunologists for almost 20 years. Although a great deal is known about the MHC of mouse and man, relatively little is known about the MHC of other species. Thus, the time seemed right to organize a conference to bring together researchers working on the MHC of domestic animal species.

These proceedings are the results of a symposium held in Ames, Iowa, October 23–24, 1987, to discuss the latest knowledge on the MHC of four domestic species: the pig, the cow, the horse, and the chicken. The two-day symposium was attended by 190 registrants from 16 countries. In addition to the nine plenary talks, 40 abstracts were presented, which included information on four other species: the dog, the cat, the sheep, and the pheasant.

We look back upon the conference as having been a great success. Many researchers in the same field were able to meet each other for the first time, and many new collaborations arose as the result of this meeting. A particular highlight of the conference was the banquet at which we presented Arne Nordskog with a plaque commemorating over 40 years of research at Iowa State and his discovery that the B blood group of the chicken was the chicken MHC. And who could forget Chella David's after-dinner talk?

We are extremely grateful to all of you who attended and to all who made this conference such a great success. We especially thank Richard Willham for drawing the animals for the logo, and Marit Nilsen-Hamilton for proposing that Iowa State sponsor a series of conferences, of which ours was the second. This conference would not have been possible without the help of the many graduate students, postdocs, technicians, and secretaries in all of our labs who worked tirelessly arranging the poster sessions, decorations, transportation, picture taking, and a host of other details that made this conference special. We hope that you find these proceedings informative and that you enjoy reading these papers as much as we did!

May 6, 1988   CAROL WARNER
                                               MAX ROTHSCHILD
                                               SUE LAMONT

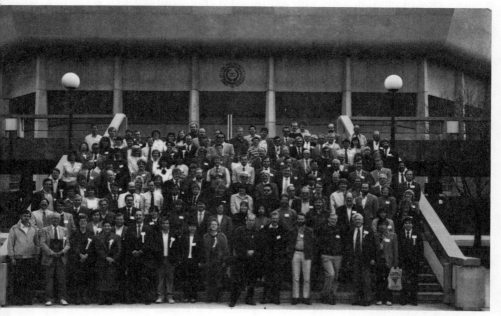

Participants at MHC conference

PART 1

Plenary Papers

Gene Expression in Chickens Aneuploid for the MHC-bearing Chromosome

S. E. Bloom, M. E. Delany, D. M. Muscarella, R. R. Dietert, W. E. Briles, and R. W. Briles

A genetic system for increasing the number of copies of the major histocompatibility complex (MHC) was developed using chickens having extra numbers (aneuploidy) of a microchromosome that also contains the ribosomal RNA genes (rRNA). We investigated the question of whether the MHC and rRNA genes are expressed in a dosage-dependent manner in aneuploids. Chickens having two, three, and four copies of the rDNA/MHC microchromosome were produced from crosses of trisomic parents. Analysis of Southern blots revealed that the rDNA copy numbers were directly proportional to the number of rDNA/MHC microchromosomes. Although RNA processing was not different, the amounts of pre-ribosomal and mature ribosomal RNAs were at diploid levels in both normal and aneuploid cells. Regulation of rRNA gene expression in aneuploid cells was shown to be achieved by inactivation of rRNA genes. In contrast, increased amounts of surface Ia molecules, encoded by the B-L MHC subregion, were detected on B-lymphocytes from aneuploids. Also, alterations in B-cell development were observed in aneuploid embryos and neonates. Thus, the MHC is expressed in a gene dosage-dependent fashion, over a range of two, three, and four copies per cell while neighboring rRNA genes are subject to inactivation.

INTRODUCTION

The major histocompatibility complex (MHC) is one of the most intriguing and biologically influential of the multigene families in animals and man (17). This complex encodes surface molecules essential for cell communication and immune surveillance systems of the body. Of high interest in animal genetics and breeding are the possibilities for enhancing resistance to various disease pathogens by detecting and utilizing variations for class I and class II MHC genes in selection programs. Extensive variations in MHC genes have already been described for the mouse (17). In addition, there is evidence to support roles for MHC and closely linked genes in regulating immune development, growth, and even reproductive fitness.

In order to fully appreciate the power and range of influence of the MHC, it is essential to understand its genetic and molecular structure as well as the

Bloom, Delany, Muscarella, and Dietert: Depts. of Poult. and Avian Sci., and Biochem., Mol. and Cell Biol., Cornell Univ., Ithaca, N.Y. Briles and Briles: Dept. of Biol. Sci., Northern Ill. Univ., De Kalb, Ill.

influence and interactions of each of its gene products. Thus, there is much activity today in cloning and sequencing MHC genes, characterizing gene arrangements within the complex, and studying regulation of expression of its genes in various cell systems. It is equally important to investigate quantitative variations in MHC-encoded molecules on the lymphocyte surface and the influence of such variations on cell-cell interactions in the context of immune development and immune functions. Studies of both human and mouse lymphocytes show a role for quantity of surface Ia antigen in regulating T-B lymphocyte interactions. For example, increases in B-cell Ia antigen lead to enhanced activation of B-cells by T-helper cells (2,6,15).

Developments in genetic engineering now allow for insertion of MHC and other genes into cells and animals. To determine whether such manipulations will be useful for animal improvement, it will be necessary to determine whether extra MHC genes are expressed in the appropriate cells, the extent of increase in cell surface molecules, and the ultimate biological outcome (beneficial versus teratogenic response) for the animal.

Studies with the Trisomic Model System

We have been able to investigate certain aspects of MHC regulation and dosage effects in vivo using a unique genetic system in the chicken. The number of MHC copies can be increased by one and by two per cell by crossing chickens trisomic for the particular MHC-bearing microchromosome. Since this small chromosome contains less than 1% of chromosomal DNA, animals with trisomic and tetrasomic (aneuploid) genotypes can be hatched out, and many reared to adult stage. Thus, alterations in development of the immune and other systems of interest can be studied in detail and related to MHC chromosome dosage and the status of gene expression.

The microchromosome involved in the aneuploidy contains the MHC but also a second major complex that encodes the 18S, 5.8S, and 28S ribosomal RNAs, namely the ribosomal RNA gene cluster (rDNA). We, therefore, investigated gene expression and regulatory mechanisms for both gene complexes in aneuploid cells. Such studies revealed that extra rRNA genes are regulated so that diploid amounts of ribosomal RNAs are present in both trisomic and tetrasomic cells. On the contrary, the MHC was found to be regulated in a dosage-dependent fashion, at least for class II genes and probably class I and class IV (B-G subregion) genes as well. Given this situation of differential expression of MHC versus rDNA genes, a unique opportunity was presented to study the effects of incremental increases in MHC products, such as Ia antigen, on immune development and functions, as well as on other non-immune biological functions.

It is the purpose of this review to present the major findings concerning regulation of expression of extra copies of MHC and rDNA genes in the trisomic model system. Our results concerning MHC dosage influences on the development of the immune and other biological systems in the chicken are also included.

The Chicken MHC: Modulation of Gene Dosage

The MHC of the chicken was discovered as a blood group system by Briles et al. (1950) and was later shown to exert strong responses in skin grafts by Schierman and Nordskog (1961). This system, designated the B complex, is now considered the phylogenetic homologue of the mammalian MHC (23). Three major subregions are known for the chicken MHC: B-L, B-F, and B-G. The former two correspond to the mammalian class II and class I regions, respectively. The latter, or class IV region, encodes erythrocyte antigens only, and it has no known mammalian counterpart (14,24). The chicken MHC is linked to the rDNA, and both gene complexes reside on a microchromosome, about 16th in size (Fig. 1) (3,4). It is estimated that some 6,000 Kb of DNA are arranged as 145 rDNA tandem repeats constituting the nucleolar organizer region (NOR) on this microchromosome (21).

MHC dosage can be modulated using two types of genetic schemes. In the first (type I), matings are made between trisomic and disomic parental types. This trisomic x disomic mating generates a 1:1 ratio of disomic and trisomic progeny in the F_1 generation. The F_1 chicks will be heterozygous for B haplotypes if parentals were heterozygotes (see Fig. 2). In the second (type II), trisomic x trisomic crosses are made, and disomic (2 MHCs), trisomics (3 MHCs), and tetrasomics (4 MHCs) chicks are produced in a 1:2:1 ratio in the F_1. As for the first mating scheme, heterozygous F_1 progeny are obtained where parentals are multiple B haplotype hetereozygotes (Fig. 4). The dosage of a particular B haplotype

can be modulated by using homozygous parents, i.e.,
a cross of $B^{15}B^{15}B^{15}$ x $\underline{B}^{15}\underline{B}^{15}\underline{B}^{15}$ parentals produces
$\underline{B}^{15}\underline{B}^{15}$, $\underline{B}^{15}\underline{B}^{15}\underline{B}^{15}$, and $\underline{B}^{15}\underline{B}^{15}\underline{B}^{15}\underline{B}^{15}$ F_1 progeny.
This latter scheme was used to study MHC dosage-
related expression on the lymphocyte surface and
dosage-dependent effects on immune development.

The genetic and molecular status of the MHC and rDNA
clusters in aneuploid animals has been established.
Quantitative Southern hybridization analyses with
cloned chicken probes for rDNA and MHC sequences
showed stepwise increases in hybridization intensity
to DNA from trisomic and tetrasomic cells, respectively (13,21).

CHROMOSOME MAPS

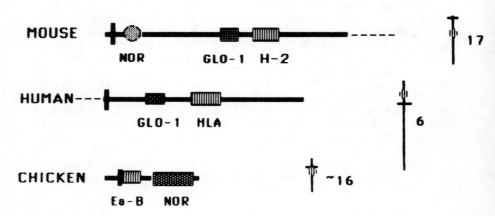

Fig. 1. Chromosomal localizations of the MHC in
mouse (H-2), human (HLA), and chicken (Ea-B). The
MHC and nucleolar organizer region (NOR) are linked
in mouse and chicken.

Each MHC Copy is Expressed in Aneuploid Cells

We examined the question of whether one or more MHC copies are inactivated in aneuploid cells using types I and II matings with heterozygous parental types. Chromosome segregation in trisomics and randomness of fertilization events (with monosomic and disomic gametes equally viable) permitted a test of MHC expression versus inactivation of copies. B-complex specific alloantisera, developed for typing the Cornell strains, were used to detect MHC expression on the erythrocyte cell surface. From the model in Fig. 2, it can be seen that six types of disomic and six types of trisomic progeny are possible from the type I mating of a $\underline{B}^6 \underline{B}^{13} \underline{B}^{15}$ trisomic and a $\underline{B}^{15} \underline{B}^{21}$ disomic. The zygotic combinations that reveal the meiotic products and fertilization events are shown with asterisks. If one MHC is not expressed in the trisomic genotype (i.e., inactivation to maintain disomic status), animals that are completely homozygous or express just two haplotypes, as shown, are expected. Analysis of such type I crosses showed that all possible meiotic products and fertilization events actually occurred (4). No homozygous $\underline{B}^{15}$ trisomics were formed, and no trisomics with two haplotypes diagnostic of inactivation were detected (Fig. 3).

In the type II cross, nine zygotic types are possible (Fig. 4) if all MHC regions are expressed in all genotypes. Such crosses revealed that all expected gametic types were actually formed and participated in fertilization events. In addition to finding trisomic chickens expressing three different $\underline{B}$ haplotypes, tetrasomics expressing four $\underline{B}$ haplotypes were detected (i.e., $\underline{B}^6 \underline{B}^{13} \underline{B}^{15} \underline{B}^{21}$) (5). No homozygous $\underline{B}^6$ or $\underline{B}^{21}$ aneuploid genotypes were found (Fig. 5). Thus, it appears that the additional MHC copies present in aneuploid types are expressed, and expression on the erythrocyte surface is high enough to be detected in standard blood typing assays.

A Duplicated MHC Subregion is Expressed In Aneuploids

Using the Briles $\underline{B}^{R8}$ recombinant, it was possible to test for the expression of extra $\underline{B}\text{-}\underline{G}$ copies. The $\underline{B}^{R8}$ recombinant chromosome contains a complete $\underline{B}\text{-}\underline{G}^{23}$ region plus a reduced $\underline{B}\text{-}\underline{G}^2$ region resulting from unequal crossing over (7,19). Crosses were made between $\underline{B}^8 \underline{B}^{R8}$ heterozygotes and $\underline{B}^{15} \underline{B}^{15} \underline{B}^{15}$ trisomics. Four genotypes are possible in the F_1, and all such progeny were found (Fig. 6). $\underline{B}^{R8} \underline{B}^{15} \underline{B}^{15}$ trisomics (typing B-G23, B-G2, B15, B15) were clearly detected indicating expression of both B-G genes from the duplicated <u>B-G</u> subregion when a minimum of four <u>B-G</u> subregions (distributed among three MHC-chromosomes) per cell were present.

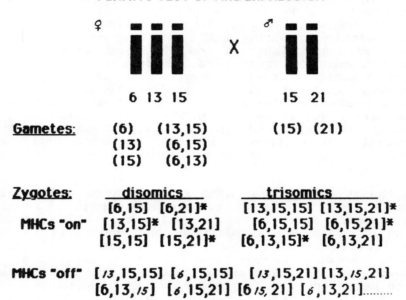

CHROMOSOME SEGREGATION IN TRISOMICS:
PERMITS TEST OF MHC EXPRESSION

♀ ▮▮▮   X   ♂ ▮▮

6 13 15   15 21

<u>Gametes:</u>   (6)   (13,15)   (15) (21)
          (13)   (6,15)
          (15)   (6,13)

<u>Zygotes:</u>   <u>disomics</u>   <u>trisomics</u>
MHCs "on"   [6,15] [6,21]*   [13,15,15] [13,15,21]*
            [13,15]* [13,21]   [6,15,15]   [6,15,21]*
            [15,15] [15,21]*   [6,13,15]* [6,13,21]

MHCs "off" [*13*,15,15] [*6*,15,15] [*13*,15,21][13,*15*,21]
            [6,13,*15*] [*6*,15,21] [6*15*,21] [*6*,13,21]........

Fig. 2. Type I cross of trisomic x disomic chickens generating a 1:1 ratio of disomic and trisomic F_1 progeny. Numbers are <u>B</u> haplotypes. Shown are haplotypes expected if all MHCs are expressed. If one or more MHC regions are inactive in trisomics, homozygotes and selected heterozygotes result. Lower case haplotypes in italics symbolize unexpressed MHC genes. The zygotic combinations that reveal the meiotic products and fertilization events are shown with asterisks.

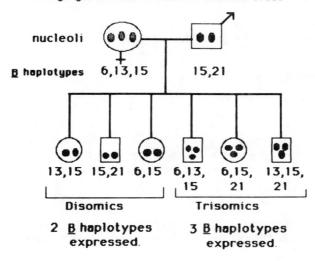

Fig. 3. Segregation and expression of MHC genes in disomic and trisomic progeny in a representative family.

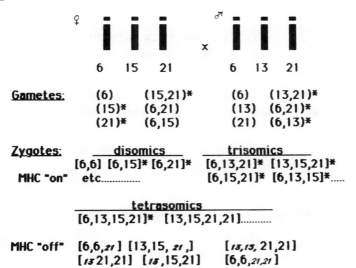

Fig. 4. Model for type II cross generating disomic, trisomic, and tetrasomic progeny. Lower case numbers in italics symbolize unexpressed MHC genes. Asterisks indicate diagnostic genetic types and examples of diagnostic zygotic types.

Detecting MHC expression in aneuploid
segregants from Trisomic x Trisomic cross

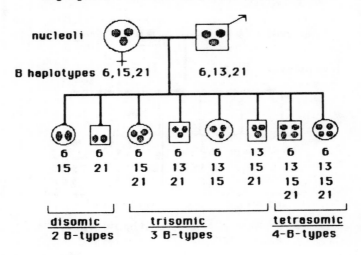

Fig. 5. Segregation and expression of MHC genes in normal and aneuploid progeny in a representative family.

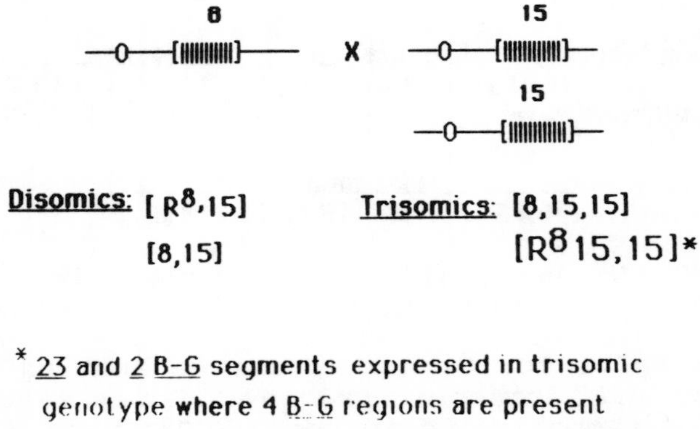

TEST FOR EXPRESSION OF SUBREGIONS
IN A B-G DUPLICATION (Briles R⁸)

R^8

23 2	15

8	15

X

| | 15 |

Disomics: [R⁸,15]

[8,15]

Trisomics: [8,15,15]

[R⁸15,15]*

* 23 and 2 B-G segments expressed in trisomic
genotype where 4 B-G regions are present

Fig. 6. Expression of extra B-G regions in trisomic segregants having the R^8 recombinant chromosome.

Extra rDNA Repeats in Aneuploids are Not Recruited for Transcription

Evidence from a number of lines indicates that rDNA genes are transcribed from each MHC/rDNA microchromosome in trisomic and tetrasomic cells (Fig. 7). This includes the findings of three and four complete and functional nucleoli in trisomic and tetrasomic cells, respectively, assessed by acridine orange cytochemistry and electron microscopy (18, 21). In addition, three and four microchromosomes are stained in trisomic and tetrasomic cells by the Ag-AS technique detecting transcriptionally active nucleolar organizers (4,12,20).

Examinations of the amounts of mature ribosomal RNA products in aneuploid cells revealed no increases above amounts measured in diploid cells despite the increases in rRNA gene copy numbers (21). No evidence of regulation at the levels of rate of transcription or RNA processing were found. Rather, regulation of gene expression was found to be operating at the chromatin level. For example, chromatin

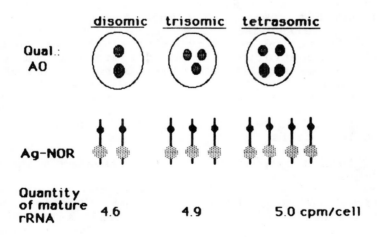

Fig. 7. Summary of gene expression for rRNA gene clusters (NORs) in aneuploids. Although all NORs are expressed, the levels of mature rRNAs are regulated to diploid amounts. Regulation is at the chromatin level. AO = acridine orange stained; Ag-NOR = silver-stained nucleolar organizer region.

from tetrasomic cells was more resistant to DNase I digestion than chromatin from disomic controls suggesting that a portion of the rRNA genes in the aneuploid cells was inactive (22).

Topoisomerase I (topo I) is specifically associated with transcriptionally active genes, and the drug camptothecin is a specific inhibitor of this enzyme. Treatment of cells with camptothecin and subsequent lysis of the cells with SDS results in single-strand breaks in the DNA at the sites of the topo I-DNA complexes (11). From the extent of cleavage of rDNA, an estimate of the number of active genes per cell was made in rapidly dividing chicken embryo fibroblasts (22). From such analysis, it appears that of the 290, 470, and 590 rDNA repeats per cell in disomic, trisomic, and tetrasomics, respectively, only about 200 genes are recruited for transcription in each genotype.

MHC-Encoded Glycoprotein is Increased on the Aneuploid Erythrocyte Surface

Using the type II mating scheme and homozygous $\underline{B}^{15}$ parental types, we examined quantitative aspects of MHC expression in aneuploid erythrocytes. Trisomic and tetrasomic erythrocytes showed increased adsorption power toward a B-15 reactive alloantiserum by 38% and 68% respectively when compared to disomic cells. Tetrasomic cells also showed greater hemagglutination capacity (agglutinated at limiting serum concentrations) than disomic control cells (9). These results indicated increased numbers of MHC encoded molecules on aneuploid erythrocytes. The alloantisera used in these studies recognized B-F but also B-G molecules. It is likely that products of both these subregions were increased on aneuploid cells.

Aneuploid B Lymphocytes Express Elevated Amounts of a Class II Product

Flow cytometry was used to measure the amounts of Ia antigen on aneuploid B-lymphocytes. Surface Ia was quantitated using the cIa-1 monoclonal antibody (10) plus a secondary FITC-labeled antibody. A stepwise increase (over diploid level) in surface Ia was detected on trisomic and tetrasomic B-cells (Fig. 8) obtained from progeny of type II trisomic matings using homozygous $\underline{B}^{15}$ parentals. These results clearly indicated dose-dependent expression of the class II genes over the range of two, three, and four MHC copies.

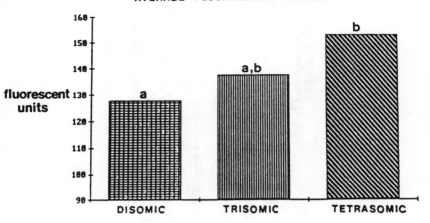

Fig.8. Surface amounts of Ia antigen on B-cells is increased incrementally in animals with two, three, or four MHC chromosomes, respectively. Values without a common letter (a, b) differ significantly (p < .01).

Differential Gene Expression on the MHC/rDNA Microchromosome

The picture that emerges from our studies of gene activity is that of two tightly linked gene complexes differentially regulated in aneuploid cells (Fig. 9). Regulation for either gene complex is not at the whole chromosome or gene complex levels. Rather, each MHC and rDNA complex is expressed at dosages of 2, 3 and 4 complex copies per cell. For the MHC, a major mode of gene regulation is MHC dosage. This mechanism is strongly supported by the studies on Ia quantitation on B-cells. A stepwise increase in this class II MHC product was detected on embryonic and neonatal B-cells in disomic, tri-somic, and tetrasomic genotypes, respectively. Gene dosage-dependent regulation was also confirmed for MHC-encoded erythrocyte glycoproteins. It remains to be determined whether the number of MHC-encoded molecules is directly proportional to the increments of gene dosage (i.e., 50% and 100%) or rather increased by smaller increments up to a tightly regulated plateau of permissible surface expression. Also, we do not yet know the status of expression of other MHC subregions.

Differential Gene Expression

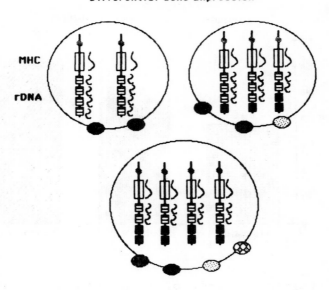

Fig. 9. Model for gene expression of the MHC and rDNA in disomic, trisomic, and tetrasomic cells. Both genetic regions are expressed, but only a subset of rRNA genes are recruited for transcription.

Regulation in rDNA expression is at the sub-complex level. While all rDNA complexes or NORs are in fact actively transcribing in aneuploid cells, not all available rRNA genes are used. Subsets of rRNA genes are recruited so that about 200 genes are transcribing in disomic, trisomic and tetrasomic cells at any one time. It is not known if gene activation occurs in blocks or "domains" of rDNA repeats or if this process is at random along the rDNA tandem.

Increased MHC Dosage is Associated with Altered Immune Development

Bursal development was found to be altered incrementally by increased MHC dosage. Trisomic and tetrasomic chicks had smaller bursae than diploids detected as early as 2 days post-hatching. The composition of the developing B-cell populations in bursae were clearly altered. Flow cytometry analysis revealed a reduction in the large cell subpopulation of the bursal resident B-cells in aneuploid embryos and chicks (10). Aneuploid embryos (18 days of incubation) had fewer B-cells expressing Ia antigen and also fewer cells expressing IgM. Such differences were less apparent in one week old chicks (Fig. 10). The development of IgG positive cells was noteworthy. Tetrasomics and trisomics showed greatly increased percentages of IgG cells at 1 week of age compared to diploid controls.

The proportion of cells in mitosis was lower in both trisomic and tetrasomic B-cell populations at 18 days of incubation and at 1 week post hatch, but not at 1 day post hatch. Taken together these results indicate a MHC dosage-related perturbation of B-cell differentiation. We speculate that this perturbation is mediated primarily by excess surface Ia present on aneuploid B-lymphocytes. The nature of the perturbation is to have an embryonic bursae deficient in 1) Ia positive cells, 2) IgM positive cells, and 3) large B-cell types, that may well be the pool of undifferentiated cells. The apparent burst of IgG production in neonates may represent a compensatory expansion of a somewhat limited set of B-cell clones developed in aneuploid embryos.

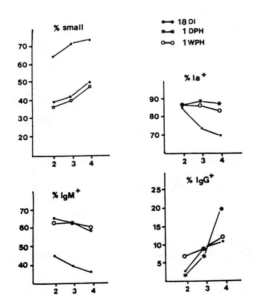

Fig. 10. Flow cytometry analysis of B-cells for sizes and expression of antigen markers. Numbers on abscissas are genotypes and on ordinates are percentages.

Wider Ranging Influences of MHC Dosage

In the propagation and maintenance of our genetic
stocks, we have detected a variety of biological
alterations associated with MHC dosage. Most notable
is the dramatic loss of tetrasomic chicks within the
first few weeks after hatching. Mortality is due to
splay legs, heart malfunctions and possibly infections. Later mortality is due primarily to Marek's
disease virus. Growth of aneuploid chicks is
reduced, slightly in trisomics but dramatically in
tetrasomics. Reproduction in females is drastically
reduced, primarily the result of deficient egg
production. Tetrasomic males, although difficult to
use in artificial insemination, are nevertheless
fertile in natural pen matings. Finally, preliminary
observations of aneuploids suggest behavioral
modifications. Obvious is the extreme shyness of
adult tetrasomics and quickness to become agitated
upon routine handling. Our findings are consistent
with other reports of MHC haplotype effects on early
development in the mouse and later growth and reproduction in animals including poultry (1,16,26). The
trisomic line of chickens should be a useful model
for the continued investigation of MHC-related
influences on developing systems, reproduction, and
behavior in animals.

SUMMARY AND CONCLUSIONS

The trisomy model system facilitated the investigation of both qualitative and quantitative aspects of
MHC regulation in the context of increases in MHC
chromosome dosage over the range of 2, 3, and 4
copies. Since the rDNA gene cluster, or NOR, is
tightly linked to the MHC, copy number variants or
aneuploids are easily detected by scoring maximum
nucleolus number per cell in embryonic tissues or in
feather pulp of chicks, growing birds and adults.
MHC dosage was modulated using type I (one parent
trisomic) and type II (both parents trisomics)
mating schemes. In the former, a 1:1 ratio of
disomic and trisomic progeny was produced. A 1:2:1
ratio of disomic:trisomic:tetrasomic progeny was
generated in the latter mating scheme.

Chromosome segregation in trisomics and randomness
of fertilization events (with viability of monosomic
and disomic gametes) permitted a test of MHC expression versus inactivation of copies. Blood typing of
progeny from type I and II matings involving heterozygous parentals revealed that all MHC regions were
expressed in trisomic (3 MHCs) and tetrasomics (4

MHCs). B-glycoprotein expression from the extra MHC copies at the cell surface is high enough to be readily detected in routine blood typing tests. Thus, we find no evidence for inactivation of MHC regions in the range of 2 to 4 copies per cell.

Using the Briles $\underline{B}^{R8}$ recombinant chromosome, it was possible to examine expression of a duplicated $\underline{B-G}$ segment of the MHC in the context of extra MHC copies. Both portions of the $\underline{B-G}$ duplication, $\underline{B}^{23}$ and $\underline{B}^2$, were expressed in the trisomic cell along with two normal $\underline{B-G}^{15}$ subregions. Here again, no inactivation of MHC genes is apparent.

Expression of the neighboring ribosomal RNA genes was examined, and like the MHC region, all rDNA clusters in aneuploid cells are expressed. However, the amount of gene product, the 18S+5.8S+28S RNAs, in aneuploid cells is regulated to diploid levels. This is achieved by recruitment of about 200 rRNA genes per cell for transcription in all genotypes.

Quantitative analysis of MHC cell surface products revealed that aneuploid erythrocytes and B-lymphocytes had increased numbers of surface molecules. The increases were correlated with the MHC dosages. Our analyses included expression of class II, class I, and probably class IV genes. Further studies are needed to dissect more clearly the respective levels of genetic activity for the various class I, IV, and possibly other MHC genes in various cell populations.

The overall model that has emerged is one involving differential gene expression of the MHC and rDNA regions on the microchromosome (Fig. 8). In aneuploid cells both genetic regions are expressed on each chromosome present. A major control for surface expression of MHC products is MHC gene dosage, at least in the range of 2 to 4 copies per cell. We found this true for erythrocytes and B-lymphocytes of the bursa. In contrast, cells recruit a subset of available rDNA genes for transcription. We estimated that about 200 rRNA genes are used in normal and aneuploid cells to generate the needed levels of mature ribosomal RNAs.

Finally, we presented evidence for MHC-related perturbations of B- cell development, growth rate, livability, reproductive fitness, and behavior. Altered B-cell development in the bursa involved

reduced proliferation index, deficiencies in the
number of large cells, and fewer Ia and IgM positive
cells.   IgG expression was aberrant with unusually
large numbers of IgG positive cells in tetrasomic
chicks. Continuing studies using the trisomic model
system should be very useful for further characterizing the contributions of the various MHC genetic
subregions to specific aspects of immune development, disease resistance, growth, and reproductive
fitness.

ACKNOWLEDGEMENTS
The authors appreciate the encouragement and helpful
discussions with Edward Buss, Douglas Gilmour, Louis
Schierman, Sue Lamont, Arne Nordskog, Robert Taylor,
Jr., and Walter Collins. Bill Harris provided
technical assistance at the Cornell Flow Cytometry
facility and Ellen Willand and Jim Putnam assisted
in the laboratory. We thank Marcia Miller for sharing some of her data on cloning and characterizing
the B-G subregion of the chicken MHC. The editorial
assistance of Diane Colf is greatly appreciated.
Supported by grants from the USDA (NY 433), Cornell
Biotechnology Program, and the NIH (ES03499).

REFERENCES
1. Bacon, L. D. 1987.   Influence of the major
    histocompatibility complex on disease resistance
    and productivity. Poultry Sci. 666:802-811.

2. Bekkhoucha, F., P. Naquet, A. Pierres, S.
    Marchetto, and M. Pierres. 1984. Efficiency of
    antigen presentation to T cell clones by (B cell
    x B cell lymphoma) hybridomas correlates
    quantitatively with cell surface Ia antigen
    expression. Eur. J. Immunol. 14:807-814.

3. Bloom, S. E.   1979.   Linkage relationships:
    Chicken.   In: Inbred and Genetically Defined
    Strains of Laboratory Animals, Part 2.   P. L.
    Altman and D. D. Katz, Ed. FASEB, Bethesda, MD.

4. Bloom, S. E., and L. D. Bacon. 1985. Linkage of
    the major histocompatibility (B) complex and the
    nucleolar organizer in the chicken: Assignment
    to a microchromosome. J. Hered. 76:146-154.

5. Bloom, S. E., W. E. Briles, R. W. Briles, M. E.
    Delany, and R. R. Dietert. 1987. Chromosomal
    localization of the major histocompatibility (B)
    complex (MHC) and its expression in chickens

aneuploid for the MHC/rDNA microchromosome. Poultry Sci. 66:782-789.

6. Bottomly, K., B. Jones, J. Kaye, and F. Jones III. 1983. Subpopulations of B cells distinguished by cell surface expression of Ia antigens. Correlation of Ia and idiotype during activation by cloned Ia-restricted T cells. J. Exp. Med. 158:265-279.

7. Briles, W. E., R. W. Briles, and R. E. Taffs. 1982. An apparent recombinant within the B-G region of the B complex. Poultry Sci. 61:1425-1426.

8. Briles, W. E., W. H. McGibbon, and M. R. Irwin. 1950. On multiple alleles affecting cellular antigens in the chicken. Genetics 35:633-652.

9. Delany, M. E., W. E. Briles, R. W. Briles, R. R. Dietert, E. M. Willand, and S. E. Bloom. 1987. Cellular expression of MHC glycoproteins on erythrocytes from normal and aneuploid chickens. Develop. Comp. Immunol. 11:613-624.

10. Delany, M. E., R. R. Dietert, and S. E. Bloom. 1988. MHC-chromosome dosage effects: Evidence for increased expression of Ia glycoprotein and alteration of B-cell subpopulations in neonatal aneuploid chickens. Immunogenetics 27:24-30.

11. Gilmour, D. S., and S. R. C. Elgin. 1987. Localization of specific topoisomerase I interactions within the transcribed region of active heat shock genes using the inhibitor camptothecin. Mol. Cell Biol. 7:141-148.

12. Goodpasture, C., and S. E. Bloom. 1975. Visualization of nucleolar organizer regions in mammalian chromosomes using silver staining. Chromosoma 53:37-50.

13. Goto, R., C. G. Miyada, S. Young, R. B. Wallace, H. Abplanalp, S. E. Bloom, W. E. Briles, and M. M. Miller. 1988. Isolation of a cDNA clone from the B-G subregion of the chicken histocompatibility (B) complex. Immunogenetics 27:102-109.

14. Hála, K., Vilhelmová, M., and J. Hartmanová. 1976. Probable crossing-over in the B blood group of chickens. Immunogenetics 3:97-104.

15. Henry, C., E. L. Chan, D. Kodlin. 1977.
    Expression and function of I region products on
    immunocompetent cells. II. I region products
    in T-B interaction. J. Immunol. 119:744-748.

16. Kim, C. D., S. J. Lamont, and M. F. Rothschild.
    1987. Genetic associations of body weight and
    immune response with the major histocompatibi-
    lity complex in White Leghorn chicks. Poultry
    Sci. 66:1258-1263.

17. Klein, J. 1986. Natural History of the Major
    Histocompatibility Complex. New York: John
    Wiley and Sons.

18. Macera, M. J., and S. E. Bloom. 1981. Ultra-
    structural studies of the nucleoli in diploid
    and trisomic chickens. J. Hered. 72:249-252.

19. Miller, M. M., Goto, R., and W. E. Briles. 1986.
    Biochemical evidence for recombination within
    the B-G region of the chicken major histocompa-
    tibility complex. Poultry Sci. 65:94.

20. Miller, O. J., D. A. Miller, V. G. Dev, R.
    Tantravahi, and C. M. Croce. 1976. Expression
    of human and suppression of mouse nucleolus
    organizer activity in mouse-human somatic cell
    hybrids. Proc. Natl. Acad. Sci. USA. 73:4531-
    4535.

21. Muscarella, D. E., V. M. Vogt, and S. E. Bloom.
    1985. The ribosomal RNA gene cluster in
    aneuploid chickens: Evidence for increased gene
    dosage and regulation of gene expression. J.
    Cell Biol. 101:1749-1756.

22. Muscarella, D. E., V. M. Vogt, and S. E. Bloom.
    1987. Characterization of ribosomal RNA
    synthesis in a gene dosage mutant: The
    relationship of topoisomerase I and chromatin
    structure to transcriptional activity. J. Cell
    Biol. 105:1501-1513.

23. Pazderka, F., B. M. Longenecker, G. R. J. Law,
    and R. F. Ruth. 1975. The major
    histocompatibility complex of the chicken.
    Immunogenetics 2:101-130.

24. Pink, J. R. L., W. Droege, K. Hála, V. C.
    Miggiano, and A. Ziegler. 1977. A three-locus

model for the chicken major histocompatibility complex. Immunogenetics 5:203-216.

25. Schierman, L. W.. and A. W. Nordskog. 1961. Relationship of blood type to histocompatibility in chickens. Science 134:1008-1009.

26. Warner, C. M. 1985. Molecular genetics and cloning of the major histocomptibility complex (MHC). Proceedings, Thirty-Fourth National Breeders' Roundtable. p. 180-202.

SLA, the Major Histocompatibility Complex in Swine: Its Influence on Physiological and Pathological Traits

M. Vaiman, Ch. Renard, and N. Bourgeaux

SLA (Swine Lymphocyte Antigen) the major histocompatibility complex of this species contains several subsets of closely linked loci, some of which are highly polymorphic. Serological testing for class-I antigens alone has so far allowed the characterization of over 60 different haplotypes. Besides constituting the strongest transplantation barrier in swine the SLA region appears to affect a variety of biological processes, some of which are of economic importance. The SLA complex has been shown to play a part in immune responses to various antigens and vaccines, and also in complement activity. Associations between the SLA complex and several reproductive traits of low heritability have been found. According to serological criteria, very similar haplotypes were observed to have a negative influence on the ovulation rate in sows and on sexual organ development in boars. Furthermore the frequency of a given haplotype in a selective hyperprolific herd was shown to increase significantly compared to the average population. Associations between the SLA complex, carcass composition and growth performances were also observed in young adults. Similarly, in piglets, viability, and weight at birth and weaning are associated with certain SLA haplotypes. Prolificacy is also affected in matings in which boars and sows have common SLA haplotypes. The mechanisms behind these associations are presently unknown although the mapping of genes already characterized inside the SLA complex (e.g. enzyme 21 hydroxylase) and the probable existence of others as yet undefined might be relevant to the numerous effects of the SLA complex.

THE SWINE lymphocyte antigen system (SLA) constitutes the major histocompatibility complex (MHC) of the Sus scrofa species. The system has been mapped on chromosome 7, close to the centromere, and is probably located on the short arm (1,2). Two blood group systems, J and C, are linked to the SLA region. The J locus is located about 10 centimorgans away from the SLA complex, and the C locus, 5 centimorgans from the J locus (3). The gene coding for the enzyme glyoxalase is probably also located close to the SLA complex (4). Lastly, the genes coding for two other enzymes, mannose phosphate isomerase and nucleoside phosphorylase, are also located on chromosome 7 (5). The nucleoside phosphorylase locus has been mapped in the middle of the long arm (Yerle , personal communication). The location of the mannose phosphate isomerase gene is not known.

As in other mammals, the major histocompatibility complex in swine comprises several subsets of closely linked genes, encompassing about one centimorgan, and each subset contributes a different family or class of molecules. So far as we know, all the functioning genes of the SLA complex appear to be codominantly expressed. At the molecular level there are 6 to 10 class I potential genes per haploid genome, which were

Vaiman: CEA-IPSN-DPS Laboratoire de Radiobiologie Appliquée 91191 Gif sur Yvette, France.
Renard and Bourgeaux: CEA-INRA Laboratoire de Radiobiologie Appliquée 78350 Jouy-en-Josas, France.

detected by a combination of Southern blotting and DNA probe hybridization (6,7). The functional class I genes code for polymorphic transmembrane glycoproteins of about 45 kilodaltons (KD). When non-covalently combined with beta-2-microglobulin, these glycoproteins constitute the SLA class I antigens. The latter are expressed by all nucleated cells and also by platelets, but not by erythrocytes.

The occurrence within litters of piglets bearing SLA class I recombined haplotypes on the one hand, and the results of lysostrip and immunocytochemical experiments on the other, have led to the conclusion that there are at least three functional SLA class I loci whose products or antigens are definable serologically (8). So far, more than 40 different SLA class I specificities have been characterized and tentatively allocated to one of the three series of SLA class I loci (A ,B or C).

Serological testing for class I antigens alone has until now allowed the characterization of more than 60 haplotypes (9). This figure is far below what can be expected considering that 8-15 alleles have been assigned to each of the above series. It is not yet clear why the known range of SLA antigenic associations is so limited.

The SLA class II gene family comprises 2-4 potentially functional alpha genes, and 8-12 beta genes per haploid genome. SLA class II products are heterodimers of a 33 KD alpha or heavy glycoprotein chain and of a 28 KD beta or light chain. Evidence exists for at least two subpopulations of SLA class II molecules, characterized as DR-like and DQ-like molecules. These molecules are expressed mainly by B cells, macrophages and certain subsets of T cells. SLA class II antigen serology is much less advanced than class I serology. Consequently, the degree of polymorphism of the class II products is not yet clear. However, when the polymorphism of the class II region was probed using homozygous typing cells in one-way mixed lymphocyte reactions, its degree of variability was significant (10).

The SLA class III region has so far been characterized through the existence of gene(s) coding for the C4 complement constituent, itself flanked by a gene coding for the enzyme 21 hydroxylase (11). The latter plays a key role in the biosynthesis of adrenal steroids, and may influence sexual steroid levels.

INFLUENCE OF THE SLA COMPLEX ON PHYSIOLOGICAL AND PATHOLOGICAL
TRAITS.

In mammals ,the MHC plays a central role in the immune
response and constitutes the strongest transplantation barrier
in man and other species. The prevalent role of the swine SLA
complex in allografts is also well documented (9). Furthermore,
in man a great variety of pathological disorders has been
found to be associated with the MHC region (12). Similarly, it
has been known for some time that in rodents the MHC complex
influences numerous physiological and pathological traits,
especially hormonal metabolism (13). Evidence was recently
obtained that the HLA complex may well be involved in the
intermediary cell metabolism. For instance, it was shown that
HLA class I antigens bind specifically to cell surface
receptors, particularly those for two peptide hormones-
epidermal growth factor and insulin, thereby probably forming
genuine compounds (14). The physiological significance of
these multichain products is not yet clear.

A whole range of observations has therefore accumulated
for man and other species, including birds, thus providing
fairly promising prospects for developing research in swine on
the possible influence of the SLA complex on performance
traits.

Because quantitative traits display physiological variations and are largely dependent upon environmental conditions,
the variations ascribable to SLA probably constitute only a
small fraction of the total. Therefore, a large panel of SLA
tested animals and above all adequate controls are needed to
arrive at results of statistical significance. These require-
ments are usually not easily fulfilled, but despite the difficulties a number of informative findings have been reported.

However, the fact that these findings were obtained by a
small number of laboratories means that many more results are
needed before any definite conclusions about the role of SLA
in zootechnical performances can be drawn.

I- Influence of the SLA complex on immune responses and
complement activity.

Genetic differences in the immune responses of swine to
antigens or vaccines have been repeatedly reported. Several
attempts have been made to correlate the immune responses to
SLA phenotypes or genotypes. A summary of these observations
is given in table 1.

TABLE 1 ASSOCIATIONS OF SLA ANTIGENS WITH IMMUNE RESPONSES AND COMPLEMENT ACTIVITY.

Antigens or Vaccines	SLA haplotype	Results	Breed	Ref
Bordetella bronchiseptica	a[a] (H10)[b]	Good responders	various breeds	(15)
(T,G)-A--L	a (H10)	Antibody producer	miniature pig	(17)
	c[a] (CR-H2)[c]	"	"	"
	d[a] (H4)[b]	non producer	"	"
	c/d[d]	"	"	"
Lysozyme (hen-egg white)	a (H10)	High responder	"	"
	d (H4)	"	"	"
	c (CR-H2)	Low responder	"	"
	H10	Low responder	Large White	(18)
	H12	High responder	"	"
	H10/H12[e]	"	"	"
Serum IgA level	H4	High level	German breeds	(19)
Mitogen response (in vitro)	H4	High response capacity	"	"
Complement activity	H10	High	Large White	(20)
	H12	Low	"	"
	H10/H12[e]	Intermediate	"	"

a : The SLA haplotypes established in three miniature swine lines by D. Sachs.(16)

b : Nomenclature code of SLA haplotypes which exhibit complete serological homology with the "a" and "d" haplotypes in miniature swine.

c : Partial serological homology between the class I antigen controlled by the "c" haplotype of the miniature line and the SLA H2 haplotype in Large White.

d : Miniature swine line bearing a recombined SLA haplotype comprising the class I "c" specificities and the "d" SLA-D region.

e : SLA heterozygous pigs.

Although multigenic control of the immune response is the rule, the results displayed in table 1 show that it is influenced by the SLA complex, even when complex antigens like Bordetella bronchiseptica are used (15). Two of the three lines of miniature swine produced by D. Sachs (16), respectively bearing the SLA "a" and "c" haplotypes, were found to respond well to the synthetic compound (T,G)-A--L, whereas swine of the "d" haplotype line were non-responders. However, the latter did exhibit a high response to Hen-egg white lysozyme (HEL) as did swine with the "a" haplotype. Pigs with the "c" haplotype exhibited no noticeable response to HEL. In addition, the experiments performed in SLA recombined miniature pigs demonstrated that the immune response against (T,G)-A--L and HEL was mainly controlled by the SLA-D or class II region (17). As shown in table 1, the observations concerning the immune response of animals with apparently similar SLA haplotypes, i.e. miniature pigs with the "a" haplotype and Large White pigs with the H10 haplotype (18), are conflicting. In fact, however, the SLA-D region of these 2 haplotypes are distinctly different, even though they have been found to be indistinguishable by serological testing. One-way mixed lymphocyte reactions between homozygous SLA "a" miniature pigs and homozygous SLA H10 Large White animals gave positive but moderate responses (results not shown). These responses indicated the existence of different class II products in both types and therefore provided clues to the behavior of their opposite immune responses.

As shown in table 1 experiments set up in vivo and in vitro to evaluate the immunocompetence profile of pigs have provided evidence for higher immune capacities in those exhibiting SLA class I H4 products (19).

As recalled in table 1, quantitative differences in complement hemolytic activity have also been correlated to SLA haplotypes. Homozygous SLA H10 Large White pigs displayed higher activity than those bearing the SLA H12 haplotype, while the activity in heterozygous H10/H12 animals was intermediate (20). Note that these results were obtained before the characterization of the genes of what has been defined as the SLA class III region.

II - SLA and production traits.

Several years ago, preliminary results were reported which suggested that some SLA haplotypes may influence carcass composition and growth rate performance (21). These results are recalled in table 2, together with those obtained from more recent investigations in groups of unrelated French Large White and Landrace females initially weighing 23-25 kilograms, which were raised in the same environment until they weighed 98-100 kilograms.

TABLE 2 : SIGNIFICANT ASSOCIATIONS BETWEEN SLA HAPLOTYPES AND PRODUCTION TRAITS.

Breeds	Large White			French Landrace				Belgian Landrace
Sex and number	Males (258)		Females (141)	Males (76)		Females (102)		Females (69)
Years of data collection	1975-1979		1986	1975-1979		1986		1980
Haplotype	H12	H6	H4	H14	H1	H4	H23	H1
Number of swine with the haplotype	24	9	35	7	11	27	25	8
Average daily weight gain(g/d)		- 92**						
Food intake index (kg Food/kg gain)		+ 0.18**						
Backfat thickness (mm)	+ 1.0*		- 2.23**	- 1.2*	+1.18*		-1.39*	+3.7**
Carcass % fat	NT		- 2.49**	NT	NT	+1.36*	-2.47***	+0.72*
Ham (kg)							+0.178*	-0.53**

NT: not tested.
*p < 0.05
**p < 0.01

As shown in table 2, these new data supply new evidence that the SLA region probably affects body composition, especially lipid metabolism. Thus , in Large White females, the SLA H4 haplotype was found to correlate with a lower-than-average fat content of the carcass. In Landrace females, however it seems to have the opposite effect . Another haplotype, SLA H23, was found to be particularly strongly correlated with carcass leanness and more weakly, although significantly, with ham development in Landrace pigs.The SLA H23 haplotype is mainly found in the latter breed. In the preliminary results referred to above significant associations were found in the French and Belgian Landrace breeds between the haplotype H1 and higher carcass fatness. In Belgian Landrace females, this haplotype was also associated with a reduction in ham weight. Since the H1 haplotype is rather uncommon in French and Belgian Landrace pigs, but is very common in Large White animals, one may wonder whether the effects observed are not caused by Large White blood admixture in both Landrace breeds.

In connection with the foregoing observations, it is worth mentioning the results of a study performed almost 20 years ago (22) by American authors. These results concerned a large scale investigation in Duroc and Hampshire pigs of the associations between pig markers, (i.e. blood groups and sero-proteins) and performance traits.

Although, few significant associations were observed, it is interesting to note that among the 12 blood groups analyzed in the Durocs, C and J were found to display certain correlations with productive traits such as the weight of individuals at 42 and 154 days, and backfat thickness.

As the loci of both these blood groups are not far from the SLA region, the observations collected 20 years ago appear to be remarkably consistent with those collected more recently in French herds. However, our own results appear to be much more significant than those observed by the American authors, even though they were obtained on a small panel. It seems justifiable to infer that typing for the SLA complex instead of for the J and C blood groups may have strengthened the link between the parameters measured and the genes affecting them. The American authors also examined the influences of the different blood markers on reproductive traits. Here again, the J and C loci showed some degree of association, although it did not reach significant levels.

III - SLA and reproductive traits.

Among the important traits in swine are those related to prolificacy. Since reproduction traits usually show poor heritability, marker systems may provide good tools for improving reproductive performances.

Compared to the dearth of results concerning performance traits, studies on the presumptive effect of the SLA complex on traits related to reproduction are relatively abundant. All the observations we know of including those which have not revealed significant associations (23) have been collected in table 3. It appears from this table that litter size at birth and weaning are at best only slightly influenced by the SLA region, with the possible exception of sows carrying the SLA H6 haplotype (24,25). Thus, in one herd, females bearing this haplotype were found to have consistently larger litters than SLA H-6 negative sows. Another study in a small group of unrelated hyperprolific sows (25) showed that the frequency of the SLA H6 haplotype was about 15 percent versus less than 5 percent in the overall population. Since this haplotype appears to influence growth performances in males negatively, (see table 1) counter selection against it may have contributed to its disappearance in one of the herds investigated (25). Several results in table 3 suggest that SLA homozygosity

TABLE 3   ASSOCIATIONS BETWEEN THE SLA COMPLEX AND PATHOLOGICAL
AND PHYSIOLOGICAL REPRODUCTIVE TRAITS

Traits	SLA typed animals	Breed	SLA haplotypes	Results (≤P)		References
1) Litter size at birth	homozygous sows	LW	H 16	negative	0.15	(24)
	sows	LW	H1,2,4,5,6[a],8 12-15-24	NS		(25)
	SLA homozygous piglets expected	LW	H 19	negative	0.10	(24)
	"	LW	all haplotypes	negative	0.05	(25)
	boars and sows[b]	LW	not determined	NS		(23)
2) Homozygotes at birth	piglets	LW	H1 H2	deficit "	0.05 0.01	(25) "
3) Litter size at weaning	sows	LW	H 19	negative	0.10	(24)
4) Piglet birth weight	sows	LW	H1	negative	0.10	(24)
	"	LR	H 23	negative	0.010	"
	piglets	LW	H 12	positive	0.10	(26)
	boars and sows[b]	LW	not determined	NS		(23)
5) Piglet weaning weight	homozygous sows	LW	H 16	negative	0.05	(24)
	sows	LW	H 23	negative	0.10	"
	"	LW	H 19	positive	0.05	"
	piglets	LW	H 12	positive	0.01	(26)
	"	LR	H7	positive	0.05	(27)
6) Piglet survival rate: before weaning after weaning	piglets "	LW LW	H1 H1	positive negative	0.05 0.01	(25) "
7) Prolificacy	sows	LW	H6	positive		(25)

Table 3 continued.

Traits	SLA typed animals	Breed	SLA haplotypes	Results	(≤P)	References
8) Ovulation rate	sows	synthetic line high ovul.rate	H10	increased frequency	0.001	(28)
			H4	decreased frequency	0.001	"
	sows	LW	H10	$25.6+0.9^d$(n5)[e]		(c)
			all-H10	18.4+4(n78)		"
			H4	18.4+2.3(n33)		"
9) Male sexual tract development	Boars	LW	H4	negative	0.01	(29)
			H15	positive	0.01	"
			H16	positive	0.01	"
10) Tissue Androstenone content	Boars	LW	H10	low	0.05	"
			H2	high	0.05	"
11) embryonic development		LW	H2	impaired	0.05	(c)
12) Segregation distortion	parents and piglets	DLR	H7	transmission 60%	0.02	(31)
13) mating failures	boars and sows[b]	LW	not determined	NS		(23)
		LW	all haplotypes	NS		(c)

a : Although not significant, sows bearing haplotype SLA H6 (10 litters) gave birth to an average of 13.2+1.0 piglets, which greatly exceeds the average mean value of 11.1+0.2 for the herd. Further, SLA H6 was unexpectedly frequent in sows characterized by consistently large litter sizes.

b : 10 SLA antigens were defined in 47 boars and 123 sows which gave rise to 424 matings.

c : unpublished data.

d : number of corpora lutea.

e : number of litters

NS : not significant

in piglets may affect litter-size negatively.

Compared to its weak influence on litter size , the SLA
complex, according to some of the results in table 3, appears
to interfere significantly during both foetal life and post-
natal development. Negative or positive effects have been
observed, depending on the haplotypes considered (24,26,27).
Thus, Landrace sows bearing the haplotype H23 had piglets
which were lighter than average at birth and to some extent at
weaning (24). It is not yet clear whether this effect is
related to the fact that , as mentioned above , the haplotype
H23 has been found to be significantly associated with
reduced carcass fatness in Landrace females. On the other
hand, piglets bearing the haplotype H12 were found to be
heavier than average at birth and even more so at weaning
(26). It should however be noted that the physiological significance of these effects is different in sows and piglets.

The still-birth rate was not found to be influenced by
the SLA complex (data not shown). In one study (table 3, ref
25), the mortality rate before weaning was lower in piglets
bearing the haplotype SLA H1, although it rose significantly
after weaning. The increased mortality in H1 piglets appeared
to be connected with a higher rate of fatal diarrhea, whose
ethiology was, however, not established (25).

In an American herd which for many generations had been
subjected to selective pressure to raise the ovulation rate,
the frequency of an SLA haplotype serologically related to the
miniature pig "a" haplotype was found to have increased
considerably compared to the control line. On the other hand,
the frequency of another haplotype resembling the miniature
pig "d" haplotype had dropped significantly (28), although a
genetic drift could not be entirely ruled out. Nevertheless,as
shown in table 3, observations in a French herd tend to support the view that the haplotype H10 (which serologically
resembles the minipig "a" haplotype) might indeed be associated with high ovulation rates. Moreover, the SLA H4 haplotype (homologous to the "d" minipig haplotype) appears to be
at best neutral regarding the ovulation rate. It is probably
no coincidence that very similar SLA H4 haplotypes were found
to affect male sexual tract development negatively (29). In
fact, testes weight in boars has been found to correlate with
the ovulation rate in closely related sows (30). Two haplotypes H15 and H16 had significant positive effects on male
genital tract development (29). The males involved were primarily selected for their high or low tissue content of androstenone, a sexual steroid compound which is a pheromone in
swine. As table 3 shows, the SLA complex did not markedly
affect the androstenone level (29).

As table 3 also indicates, matings in which boars and sows had identical SLA haplotypes occasionally gave smaller litters than matings between fully SLA-disparate parents (24,25). SLA segregation distortion has been reported in Landrace pigs (31). Finally, no correlation could be established between SLA markers and mating failures (23,c).

In matings involving, in particular, the SLA H2 haplotype, litter size reduction was combined with a significant reduction in the number of SLA H2 homozygous piglets at birth, compared to the number expected. A gamete selection mechanism during fertilization, or a higher mortality rate in pregnancies involving SLA H2 homozygous embryos, might both account for this observation. The results (table 4) of an investigation of the development rate and of embryonic loss before day 35 of gestation in groups with or without the expected SLA H2 homozygous embryos suggested that the most likely explanation was a higher mortality rate in the group with SLA H2 homozygous embryos. The data analyzed in table 4 were obtained from planned matings, carried out in a Large White herd, between generations 14 and 17 of a long-term experiment of selection for reproduction performance. As indicated in this table, a significant reduction of embryonic development was found in the group with SLA H2 homozygous embryos from the 31st day of gestation onwards. More important was the finding that the percentage of embryo loss at day 35 was twice that observed in the group without SLA H2 homozygous embryos. Before day 30, however, there was no significant difference between the two groups. A simple calculation shows that the higher mortality rate found in the group with SLA H2 homozygous foetuses may alone account for the litter size reduction noted at birth. Therefore, it appears that no further selective losses occurred after day 35 of gestation. Although the precise mechanism responsible for the greater losses in the SLA H2 homozygous group is not known, the existence of recessive lethal genes within the SLA region can be suggested.

TABLE 4 : INFLUENCE OF THE SLA H2 HAPLOTYPE ON EMBRYONIC DEVELOPMENT AND LITTER SIZE.

Mating type	Embryonic development (31+32 days)				30-35 days	Litter size at birth (n)	H2/H2 piglets at birth (%)
	Placenta weight (g)	Amniotic fluid (ml)	Embryo weight (g)	Embryo length (mm)	Embryo loss (%)		
boars sows							
H2^a/--x H2/-	27.8*(70)^b	171*	1.76*	25.9*	35.5^{*c}(17)^d	9.86±1.1*(6)^c	9^{*f}
H2/-x -/-^{e}	43.5(59)^b	208	2.69	29.2	19.8^c(27)^d	12.75± 0.7(12)^c	

* P < 0.05.
a : the SLA H2 haplotypes found in the boar and sows were of the same origin. b : number of embryos. c : embryos found at 30-35 days compared to the number of corpora lutea. d : number of litters. e : control groups. f : instead of 25% expected.

CONCLUDING REMARKS

In livestock, it seems unrealistic - apart from rare cases - to expect strong correlations between any gene marker - in this case the SLA complex - and performance traits. Firstly, as already discussed above, any such correlations are likely to be of low intensity. Secondly, the exertion of selective pressures for many generations, such as those to which farm animals have obviously been subjected has led to the elimination of most of the mutations responsible for grossly harmful defects.

However, the fact that the SLA region seems to be associated with a large number of traits is particularly encouraging for the development of future research. Furthermore the role of the SLA complex in acquired and innate immunity should not be overlooked. High grade zootechnical performance depends upon many parameters, of which health status is obviously crucial. This status will particularly benefit from optimal immune responses to vaccinations and natural parasite infections. Therefore the capacity to elicit optimal immune response is of particular importance, especially in the light of the probable future large-scale use of the new vaccines. Since these vaccines are likely to be less complex than the antigenic material currently administered, and since the importance of antigen presentation is now better understood, the variability of SLA class I and class II genes might be worth taking into account in selective pig breeding. Similarly, the role of complement, especially of the constituent C4, in regulating the humoral immune response should not be overlooked.

It is too early to decide whether the SLA complex will be an important marker in future selection programs. The SLA region appears to have an appreciable effect on certain production traits. Even more important, the SLA region displays strong relationships with the ovulation rate, male sexual organ development, and piglet growth, and therefore it may well eventually become a useful tool for increasing prolificacy in swine. Similarly since piglet SLA homozygosity is quite often associated with a reduction in litter size, matings leading to such piglets should preferably be avoided. Furthermore, at birth and at weaning, SLA homozygous piglets tend to be slightly smaller than their non-homozygous littermates. Therefore, although the difference is usually not significant, SLA homozygous piglets may constitute a population of lesser fitness.

The mechanisms behind the effects of the SLA region on performance traits are presently unknown. The interesting point is that some traits appear to be related, suggesting a common origin. For example, haplotype H4 was found to be associated in Large White with carcass composition, a medium or low ovulation rate and limited male sexual organ development.

Many of these associations, or similar ones, have been described in relation to the mouse MHC, thus supporting our belief that the observations made in pig are not merely circumstantial. The mapping of genes already characterized inside the SLA complex, like the gene coding for 21 hydroxylase, and the probable existence of others which have yet not been defined, might be relevant to the variety of effects already observed for the SLA complex.

ACKNOWLEDGEMENTS

The authors wish to express their thanks to M. Dreyfus for her help in the preparation of the manuscript. We are grateful to I. Chifflet for her straightforward secretarial work.

1. Geffrotin, Cl., Popescu, C.P., Cribiu, E.P., Boscher, J.,
    Renard, Ch., Chardon, P. and Vaiman, M. 1984. Assignment
    of MHC in swine to chromosome 7 by in situ hybridization
    and serological typing. Ann. Genet.27:213-219.

2. Rabin, M. Fries, R. Singer, D. and Ruddle F.H. 1985.
    Assignment of the porcine major histocompatibility complex
    to chromosome 7 by in situ hybridization. Cytogenet. Cell
    Genet.39:206-209.

3. Hradecky, J., Hruban, V., Pazdera, J. and Klaudy, J. 1982.
    Map arrangement of the SLA chromosomal region and the J
    and C blood group loci in the pig. Anim. Blood Grps. and
    Biochem. Genet. 13:223-224.

4. Lie, W.R. Rothschild, M.F. and Warner, C.M. 1985. Quanti-
    tative differences in GLO enzyme levels associated with
    the MHC of miniature swine. Anim. Blood. Grps. and
    Biochem. Genet. 16:243-248.

5. Christensen, K., Kaufmann, U., and Avery, B. 1985. Chromo-
    some mapping in domestic pigs (Sus Scrofa) : MPI and NP
    located to chromosome 7. Hereditas. 102:231-235.

6. Satz, L.M., Wang, L-C., Singer, D.S., and Rudikoff, S.
    1985. Structure and expression of two porcine genomic
    clones encoding class I MHC antigens. J. Immunol.
    135:2167-2175

7. Chardon, P., Vaiman, M., Kirszenbaum, M., Geffrotin, Cl.,
    Renard, Ch., and Cohen, D. 1985. Restriction fragment
    length polymorphism of the major histocompatibility
    complex of the pig. Immunogenetics. 21:161-171.

8. Vaiman, M., Chardon, P., and Renard, Ch. 1979. Genetic
    organization of the pig SLA complex. Studies on nine
    recombinants and biochemical and lysostrip analysis.
    Immunogenetics. 9:353-361.

9. Vaiman, M. Histocompatibility systems in pigs. Prog. Vet.
    Microbiol. Immunol. 4. Basel. Karger. (in press).

10. Vaiman, M., Renard, Ch., Chardon, P., Garin, B., Leveziel,
    H. 1982. The D-Dr region of the pig SLA complex/analysis
    by serological and histogenetic methods. 18th Internatio-
    nal Conference on Animal Blood Groups and Biochemical
    Polymorphisms. Ottawa,Canada,July 18-24. p.15.

11. Chardon, P., Geffrotin, Cl., and Vaiman, M. Genetic
    organization of the SLA complex. (These Proceedings)

12. Ryder, L.P. and Svejgaard, A. 1981. Genetics of HLA disease association. Ann. Rev. Genet. 15:169-187.

13. Ivanyi, P. 1978. Some aspects of the H-2 system, the major histocompatibility system in the mouse. Proc. R. Soc. Lond B 202:117-158.

14. Kittur, D., Shimizu, Y., DeMars, R., and Edidin, M. 1987. Insulin binding to human B lymphoblasts is a function of HLA haplotype. Proc. Natl. Acad. Sci. USA. 84:1351-1355.

15. Rothschild M.F., Chen H.L., Christian, L.L., Lie, W.R, Venier, L., Cooper, M., Briggs, C., and Warner C.M. 1984. Breed and swine lymphocyte antigen haplotype differences in agglutination titers following vaccination with B. bronchiseptica. J. Anim. Sci. 59:643-649.

16. Sachs, D.H., Leight, G., Cone, J., Schwarz, S., Stuart, L., and Rosenberg S. 1976. Transplantation in miniature swine. I. Fixation of the major histocompatibility complex. Transplantation. 22:559-567.

17. Lunney, J.K., Vanderputten, D., and Pescovitz, M.D. 1984. MHC-linked immune response gene control of humoral and cellular responses to (T,G)-A--L and lysozyme in miniature swine. Federation Proceeding. 43:1821.

18. Vaiman, M., Metzger, J-J., Renard, Ch., and Vila, J-P. 1978. Immune response gene(s) controlling the humoral anti-lysozyme response (Ir-Lys) linked to the major histocompatibility complex SL-A in the pig. Immunogenetics.7:231-238.

19. Buschmann, H., Krausslich, H., Herrmann, H., Meyer, J. and Kleinschmidt, A. 1985. Quantitative immunological parameters in pigs - experiences with the evaluation of an immunocompetence profile. Z. Tierzuchtg. Zuchtgsbiol. 102:189-199.

20. Vaiman, M., Hauptmann, G., and Mayer, S. 1978. Influence of the major histocompatibility complex in the pig (SLA) on serum haemolytic complement levels. J. of Immunogenet. 5:59-65.

21. Capy, P., Renard, Ch., Sellier, P. et Vaiman, M. 1981. Etude préliminaire des relations entre le complexe majeur d'histocompatibilité (SLA) et des caractères de production chez le porc. Ann. Génét. Sél. Anim. 13:441-446.

22. Jensen, E.L., Smith, C., Baker L.N., and Cox, D.F. 1968.
     Quantitative studies on blood group and serum protein
     systems in pigs. II effects on production and reproduc-
     tion. J. Anim. Sci. 27:856-862.

23. Willis, G.L., Baglin, M.J., Love, R.J., Brown, S.C.,
     Nicholas, F.W. 1985. A study of histo-incompatibility and
     reproductive performance in pigs. Vet. Record. 117:601.

24. Gautschi, C., Gaillard, C., Schwander, B., and Lazary,
     S.1986. Studies on possible associations between the major
     histocompatibility complex and reproduction traits in
     swine. 3rd world congress on genetics applied to Livestock
     production, 12:70-75. Lincoln, Nebraska, USA. Dickerson,
     G.E., Johnson, R.K. eds.

25. Renard, Ch., Bolet, G., Dando, P., Vaiman, M. 1985. Rela-
     tions d'un marqueur génétique, le complexe majeur d'histo-
     compatibilité, avec la prolificité des truies et la morta-
     lité des porcelets. J. Rech. Porcine en France. 17:105-112.

26. Rothschild, M.F., Renard, C., Bolet, G., Dando, P.,
     Vaiman, M. 1986. Effect of swine lymphocyte antigen haplo-
     types on birth and weaning weights in pigs. Anim. Gene-
     tics. 17:267-272.

27. Kristensen, B., Wafler, P., de Weck, A.L. 1980. Histocom-
     patibility antigens (SLA) in swine. Possible correla-
     tion between SLA haplotypes and performance of piglets.
     Anim. Blood Grps and Biochem. Genet. 11:58-59. supp.1

28. Rothschild, M.F., Zimmerman, D.R., Johnson, R.K., Venier,
     L.,and Warner,C.M. 1984. SLA haplotype differences in
     lines of pigs which differ in ovulation rate. Anim. Blood
     Grps and Biochem. Genet. 15:155-158.

29. Rothschild, M.F., Renard, C., Sellier, P., Bonneau, M.,
     and Vaiman, M. 1986. Swine lymphocyte antigen (SLA) haplo-
     type effects on male genital tract development and andros-
     tenone level. 3rd World congress on genetics applied to
     Livestock production. 11:197-202. Lincoln, Nebraska, USA.
     Dickerson, G.E., Johnson, R.K., eds.

30. Schinckel, A., Johnson, R.K., Pumfrey, R.A., and
     Zimmerman, D.R. 1983. Testicular growth in boars of
     different genetic lines and its relationship to reproduc-
     tive performance. J. Anim. Sci. 56:1065-1076.

Genomic Hybridizations of Bovine Major Histocompatibility Genes

Leif Andersson

The genetic organization and polymorphism of bovine MHC class I and class II genes have been investigated by genomic hybridizations utilizing human probes. The human class I cDNA probe cross-hybridized strongly to bovine DNA. A complex and highly polymorphic restriction fragment pattern was obtained. The relationship to serological typing as well as the possibilities to do class I typing with DNA methods are discussed. The presence of bovine DQα, DQβ, DRα, DRβ, DOβ, DYα, DYβ, and DZα class II genes were revealed using human probes. The assessment of the number of different bovine class II genes was facilitated by the use of exon-specific probes. A striking observation was the finding that the number of DQ genes varies between haplotypes. Restriction fragment length polymorphisms (RFLPs) have been detected for all the bovine class II genes. The DQα, DQβ, and DRβ patterns were highly polymorphic. The use of the RFLP method for routine typing of class II polymorphism is discussed. The linkage relationships in the MHC region were investigated. Two additional RFLP markers, C4 and TCP1B, were also included in the analysis. The results indicated the presence of two groups of linked loci. One group comprises class I, C4, DQα, DQβ, DRα, and DRβ genes while the other comprises DOβ, DYα, DYβ, and TCP1B genes. No recombinant was observed within any of these groups of genes and there was a strong or fairly strong linkage disequilibrium between genes within groups. In contrast, a fairly high recombination frequency, about 17%, was found in the interval between the two groups of genes. The organization of the bovine MHC region is discussed in relation to the corresponding regions in other mammalian species.

THE MAJOR HISTOCOMPATIBILITY COMPLEX (MHC) of cattle is denoted BoLA for bovine lymphocyte antigens. One class I locus (BoLA-A) has been established by serological studies (1,2) while evidence for a bovine class II region (BoLA-D) was obtained by studies on the genetic control of mixed lymphocyte reactions (MLR,3). Close linkage between BoLA-A and BoLA-D has been reported (4).

When the present investigation started, about three years ago, there was virtually no information available concerning the organization of bovine MHC genes. At that time a number of MHC genes had already been cloned and well characterized in other species like man and mouse. Therefore we decided to utilize heterologous MHC probes for Southern blot analysis of genomic DNA in cattle. This paper summarizes the results obtained in a series of studies on this subject (5,6,7,8,9,10, Lindberg et al. in preparation). Our major interest has focused on the organization of the bovine class II region. We have

Dept. of Anim. Breed. and Genet., Swedish Univ. of Agric. Sci., Biomed. Ctr., Box 596, S-751 24 Uppsala, Sweden.

also investigated in detail the restriction fragment
length polymorphism (RFLP) of class II genes in order
to establish a method for routine typing of MHC class
II polymorphism in cattle. More limited studies have
been carried out on class I genes. We have also
analyzed some non-MHC genes which are known to be
linked to the MHC in other species. Finally, we have
investigated the linkage relationships in the BoLA
region by family segregation analysis and by analysis
of linkage disequilibrium.

Southern blot analysis of class I genes

A human class I cDNA probe was used to investigate
bovine class I genes by Southern blot analysis
(Lindberg et al. in preparation); the probe
corresponded to the 3' part of the gene starting from
the middle of the exon encoding the second
extracellular domain. Hybridizations of this probe to
genomic cattle DNA, digested with PvuII, resolved a
complex and highly polymorphic restriction fragment
pattern. Different individuals showed between 10 and
20 restriction fragments and only about five fragments
were constant in the material. The result is
consistent with the presence of a large number, at
least 10, of bovine class I genes.

The inheritance of class I RFLPs was investigated by
family studies. Five sire half-sib families of the
Swedish red and white breed (SRB) comprising the five
bulls, 48 different dams, and 50 offspring, were
analyzed. The interpretation of RFLPs was complicated
due to the large number of restriction fragments and
the extensive polymorphism. However, it was evident
that RFLP pattern types, composed of several variable
fragments, could be determined on the basis of the
segregation in families. The RFLP types were found to
be inherited as a distinct unit and there was no
indication of recombination between variable
fragments. No less than 21 different class I RFLP
types could be distinguished in this limited material
comprising 53 parental animals only.

The class I polymorphism was also investigated using
conventional serological tests. This test involved
sera corresponding to four internationally recognized
class I specificities (w2, w6, w10, and W16) as well
as three locally defined specificities (SRB1, SRB2,
and SRB3). A very good correlation between the

serological typing and the RFLP typing was observed. Five of the serological specificities (w2, w10, w16, SRB1, and SRB3) were found to be inherited in association with a single RFLP type in this material while the other two (w6 and SRB2) were each associated with three different RFLP types. No RFLP type was associated with more than one serological specificity.

The results show that RFLP typing could be used to study class I polymorphism in cattle. The method may be a valuable complement to conventional serological typing. For instance, it could be applied when serological typing is not feasible because fresh blood samples are not available.

The organization of the class II region

The organization of the bovine class II region was investigated by genomic Southern blot analysis (6,7,8,9). Human probes corresponding to DQα, DQβ, DRα, DRβ, DPα, DPβ, DOβ, and DZα genes were employed. The study was carried out with the aim to investigate the presence, and the number of different class II genes in the bovine genome. Southern blot analysis may be used to estimate the copy number of a given gene in the genome, provided that the following complications are taken into account. Firstly, a given restriction enzyme may cut within the hybridizing region of the probe which means that a single gene will be represented by two or more restriction fragments. In our study we have used very short (about 200 base pair long) exon-specific probes as well as multiple restriction enzymes to deal with this problem. Secondly, multiple fragments representing a single gene may be obtained due to RFLP heterozygosity. This complication was controlled by carrying out extensive family studies in order to determine the segregation patterns of variable fragments. Thirdly, the interpretations may be complicated due to cross-hybridization between closely related genes. In our study there was no problem with cross-hybridization for the α -genes but there was a problem for the β -genes. The cross-hybridizations were interpreted by comparing the relative hybridization intensities obtained with different probes. Furthermore, the use of exon-specific probes as well as multiple enzymes clearly facilitated these interpretations.

The DQ subregion. Clear evidence for the presence of bovine DQ genes was obtained. Interestingly, the

number of DQ genes was found to vary among haplotypes
(6). One group of haplotypes possesses single DQα and
DQβ genes whereas both these genes are duplicated in
the other group of haplotypes. This finding was
verified by experiments involving several restriction
enzymes, and using cDNA as well as exon-specific
probes.

The DR subregion. The results were consistent with a
single bovine DRα gene (6). Experiments with a probe
corresponding to a human DRβ 2nd domain exon indicated
the presence of at least three bovine DRβ genes.
However, a lower number of genes was indicated using a
1st domain probe. This result implies either that some
of the bovine DRβ genes lack the 1st domain exon (and
are then most likely pseudogenes) or that the human
probe did not cross-hybridize to the 1st domain exon
of some bovine DRβ genes at the stringency conditions
employed.

The DOβ and DZα genes. Human DOβ and DZα probes both
cross-hybridized well with cattle DNA (6,9). The
results clearly indicated the presence of single
bovine DOβ and DZα genes.

The DYα and DYβ genes. Two odd bovine class II genes
were recently identified (9). They were designated DYα
and DYβ since their relationship to human class II
genes is not clear. (It should be noted that they are
both denoted DY although we have no data indicating
that they are associated like DQα and DQβ genes.) DYα
and DYβ cross-hybridized primarily with the human DQα
and DRβ probes, respectively, but with a weaker
intensity than the presumed bovine DQα and DRβ genes.
They were both identified as unique class II sequences
by the finding of RFLPs which did not correlate with
DQ, DR polymorphism.

Restriction fragment length polymorphism of class II
genes.

RFLPs of bovine class II genes have been investigated
by family segregation analysis. Five sire half-sib
families of the SRB breed were analyzed. The material
comprised, besides the bulls, 48 dams and 50
offspring. As shown in Table 1, RFLPs have been
revealed for each of the different bovine class II
genes. The number of variants indicated in the table
refers to all variants detected in the family material
and in a population sample of about 200 breeding bulls
of the SRB breed. The DZα gene was in fact monomorphic

Table 1. Restriction fragment length polymorphism
of bovine class II loci.

Locus	Enzyme used	Poly morphism	No. of variants	Reference
DQα	BamHI	yes	7	7
	EcoRI	yes	5	7
	PvuII	yes	10	7,10
	TaqI	yes	19	10
	Total		20	
DQβ	BamHI	yes	10	7
	EcoRI	yes	10	7
	PvuII	yes	14	7,10
	TaqI	yes	14	10
	Total		17	
DRα	BamHI	no	–	8
	EcoRI	no	–	8
	PvuII	yes	5	8,10
	TaqI	yes	2+2	10
	Total		5	
DRβ	BamHI	no	–	8
	EcoRI	yes	2	8
	PvuII	yes	2+2	8,10
	TaqI	yes	25	10
	Total		25	
DOβ	EcoRI	no	–	6
	PvuII	yes	2	6
DZα	PvuII	no	–	9
	TaqI	yes	2	9
DYα	TaqI	yes	2	9
DYβ	PvuII	yes	2	9
	TaqI	yes	3	9

in the SRB breed but an RFLP was recently detected in
a sample representing the American Holstein-Friesian
breed analyzed in collaboration with Dr. C.J.Davies.

Limited polymorphism was revealed for DRα, DOβ, DZα,
DYα, and DYβ. The inheritance of these simple RFLPs
was confirmed by family studies.

Complex and highly polymorphic restriction fragment
patterns were obtained with each enzyme used, for both

DQα and DQβ. As already stated, this polymorphism is partly due to a variation in gene number. Careful examinations of the family data made it possible to identify different fragment pattern types. These pattern types (or RFLP types) are composed of one to four variable fragments and they segregated as alleles in this material. There was a very strong correlation between the results obtained with different enzymes. Furthermore, there was an extremely strong correlation between DQα and DQβ types. There were only a few rare exceptions to the rule that a given DQα type is always associated with the same DQβ type. An allelic series of about 20 DQ haplotypes was established on the basis of these results. These DQ haplotypes can be distinguished using two probes (DQα and DQβ) and two enzymes (PvuII and TaqI).

DRβ RFLPs were first investigated using the enzymes BamHI, EcoRI, and PvuII (8). This analysis resolved very limited polymorphism. Quite surprising, when a fourth enzyme, TaqI, was employed an extensive polymorphism was revealed (10). The number of DRβ variants in fact exceeds the number of DQα and DQβ variants as indicated in Table 1. However, the DRβ polymorphism is more difficult to type partly because the pattern is derived from multiple DRβ genes. Furthermore, most DRβ pattern types share several variable fragments with other DRβ types whereas a given DQα and DQβ type more often possess unique fragments. The fact that very limited polymorphism was revealed with other enzymes implies that the extensive TaqI polymorphism is due to restriction site polymorphism and not so-called length polymorphism (i.e. insertions, duplications etc.). The high level of polymorphism revealed using TaqI may be explained by the fact that the recognition sequence of this enzyme involves the doublet CpG. It has previously been reported that restriction sites containing CpG show a high frequency of polymorphism (11). Furthermore, it is well known that the CpG doublet occurs at a high frequency in the 5' part of variable class I and class II MHC genes (12).

RFLP typing of DQα, DQβ, DRβ, and DYα genes has also been carried out without using family information, in a population sample of about 200 breeding bulls of the SRB breed (10). This study clearly showed that the interpretations of RFLP types firmly established in the family study could be used as a key when typing unrelated animals. The genotype of virtually all individuals could be determined with confidence. The very few exceptions (one or two) were individuals which apparently were heterozygous for very rare haplotypes.

Southern blot analysis of some MHC-linked genes

The genes encoding complement components C2, C4, and Bf are located between the class I and class II region in both mouse and man. In order to test the possibility that complement component genes are located also in the bovine MHC, a full length human cDNA probe was used to screen for C4 RFLP in cattle. Genomic blots were carried out using the enzymes PvuII and TaqI, and a simple two-allele TaqI RFLP was revealed (9).

The mouse t complex constitutes a large chromosomal segment linked to the major histocompatibility complex (13). Quite recently, some cDNA clones of a gene encoding t complex polypeptide 1 (TCP1) were isolated (14). These clones were used in Southern blot analysis to study the corresponding bovine genes (5). Excellent cross-hybridization was obtained and the probes apparently hybridized to at least two bovine TCP1 genes. Two independent RFLPs, each composed of two allelic variants, were detected. One of the RFLPs, designated TCP1A, was revealed with TaqI. The other one, designated TCP1B, was evidently due to a gene duplication and was revealed with any enzyme used.

Linkage relationships in the bovine MHC region

It has previously been reported that the class I region (BoLA-A) and the class II region (BoLA-D) are closely linked (4). Close linkage between BoLA-A and blood group locus M has also been found (15).

We have utilized RFLP data on class I genes, class II genes (DQα, DQβ, DRα, DRβ, DOβ , DYα, and DYβ), C4, and TCP1B to investigate the linkage relationships in the bovine MHC region (7,8,9, Lindberg et al. in preparation). Information was also available on blood group locus M. The linkage relationships were analyzed by family segregation analyses and by analysis of linkage disequilibrium. The results clearly indicated that all these tested loci belong to the same linkage group.

The current status of the BoLA linkage group is summarized in Figure 1. It should be noted that very little information is yet available on the order of genes (see below). The map has therefore been drawn in

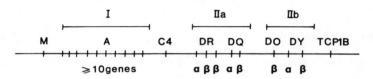

Figure 1. Genetic map of the BoLA linkage group.

accordance with the corresponding regions in man and
mouse (16,17,18) since all data available so far in
cattle are consistent with the map order in man and
mouse. Very close linkage was indicated among the M,
C4, class I, DQα, DQβ, DRα, and DRβ loci. No
recombinant in this interval was detected among 45
informative offspring and strong linkage
disequilibrium occurs among these loci. In particular,
the linkage disequilibrium in the DQ-DR region is
extremely strong. Evidence for close linkage and
significant linkage disequilibrium among the DOβ, DYα,
DYβ, and TCP1B loci were also obtained.

Surprisingly, a fairly high recombination frequency
was found between the DQ, DR class II genes and the
DO, DY class II genes (9). As many as five
recombinants among 29 informative offspring in three
different families were found, giving a recombination
estimate of 0.17 ± 0.07. The data clearly showed that
the M, C4, and class I loci map more closely to the
DQ, DR genes while the TCP1B locus maps closer to the
DO, DY genes. To indicate the subdivision of the
class II region, the DQ, DR subregion and the DO, DY
subregion are denoted IIa and IIb, respectively, in
Figure 1.

At present we have no family segregation data on the linkage relationships of DZα and TCP1A.

Discussion

Organization of the class II region. On the basis of the results of Southern blot analysis we have estimated that the bovine class II region involves one to two DQα and DQβ genes, at least three DRβ genes, and single DRα, DOβ, DZα, DYα, and DYβ genes. Thus, there are at least four α and six β class II genes in the bovine genome. This number is even higher in those haplotypes which carry duplicated DQα and DQβ genes. The results imply that the complexity of the class II region in cattle, at the genomic level, is comparable to the one in man and slightly higher than the one in the mouse. However, it is not yet known how many of the bovine genes are expressed at the protein level.

A very interesting observation was the finding of a polymorphism in the number of DQ genes among haplotypes. The observed duplication (or deletion) divides DQ haplotypes into two groups, one group possessing single DQα and DQβ genes whereas the other group possesses two pairs of DQ genes. An important question is whether the additional DQ genes are expressed at the protein level. If they are, this may have an effect on the immune response since individuals carrying duplicated DQ genes should exhibit a more extensive repertoire of DQ molecules on antigen presenting cells.

Further research is also needed to clarify the relationship between the bovine DY genes and class II genes in other species. The cloning and characterization of these genes should be straightforward.

High recombination frequency between class II subregions. The finding of a high recombination frequency between the DQ, DR and DOβ, DYα, DYβ genes in cattle was unexpected considering data on the human and murine class II region. The molecular distance between I-Aβ (the murine homologue of DQβ) and I-Aβ2 (the murine homologue of DOβ) has been determined by cosmid cloning to be about 20 kb only (18). The corresponding distance in man has been estimated to be less than 200 kb by pulsed-field electrophoresis (17). The recombination frequency in this interval is not more than 0.1% in mice (18) and not more than 3% in humans (17). Thus, the present estimate of about 17%

in cattle is strikingly different. The finding is either explained by a much larger molecular distance between these loci in cattle or by the presence of a recombination "hot spot". This question could be answered for instance by estimating the molecular distance between DQ and DOβ genes by pulsed-field electrophoresis.

Strong linkage disequilibrium in the DQ-DR region
Perhaps the most striking observation in the present investigation was the extremely strong linkage disequilibrium in the DQ-DR region. This feature was apparent with the polymorphism detected with different restriction enzymes as well as with different probes. As shown in Table 1, we have so far detected 20 DQα, 17 DQβ, 5 DRα, and 25 DRβ variants. If these variants were randomly associated they could form 42,500 different DQ-DR haplotypes. However, only about 30 have been found so far in the SRB breed, despite the fact that more than 300 animals have been RFLP-typed. The constancy of DQ-DR haplotypes was further emphasized recently when we analyzed 25 animals of the American Holstein-Friesian breed in collaboration with Dr. C.J.Davies. In this selected material we could distinguish 11 different DQ-DR haplotypes. Eight of these were apparently RFLP-identical to haplotypes in the SRB breed. Furthermore, the three remaining haplotypes previously were very similar to haplotypes found previously in the SRB breed.

Interestingly, the very low recombination frequency and the very strong linkage disequilibrium indicated in the bovine DQ-DR region is consistent with the situation in the corresponding class II region in both man and mouse (16,18). The fact that this feature has been maintained in at least three different mammalian species strongly suggests that it may be functionally important. If there is interaction with regard to fitness between alleles at different loci, Fisher (19) postulated as early as 1930 that natural selection will favour decreased recombination between these loci because it reduces the randomization pressure caused by recombination. If linkage is sufficiently tight among such gene combinations, then the complex of alleles may segregate as a single "supergene". It is quite possible that DQ-DR haplotypes should be considered as such "supergenes". This view is in fact supported by gene transfer experiments in the mouse. Cotransfection of haplotype-matched Aα and Aβ alleles (homologous to DQα and DQβ) gave good levels of class II expression at the cell surface whereas haplotype-mismatched pairs gave little or no expression (20).

RFLP typing can be used for routine typing of class II polymorphism in cattle. We have documented RFLPs for bovine DQα, DQβ, DRα, DRβ, DOβ, DZα, DYα, and DYβ genes. The inheritance of this polymorphism has been documented in all cases except for DZα. An interesting question is whether RFLP typing could be used to study class II polymorphism in unrelated animals i.e. when no family information is available. It is obvious that this could be done for DRα, DOβ, DZα, DYα, and DYβ, since these RFLPs are all very simple and involve only a small number of variants. With regard to the more complicated and more informative DQα, DQβ, and DRβ genes, allelic series of fragment pattern types were established by family analysis. These RFLP types are each composed of a particular combination of variable restriction fragments. Our studies on a population sample of 200 breeding bulls, clearly showed that RFLP typing could successfully be applied on the population level. The strong association between DQα, DQβ, and DRβ polymorphism is extremely important for the successful use of RFLP-typing.

An important topic for future research is to relate the class II polymorphism detected by RFLP-typing with that expressed at the protein level. We have recently carried out a study in collaboration with Dr. C.J.Davies to address this question. RFLP typing was performed on a sample of 25 animals of the American Holstein-Friesian breed in which class II polymorphism had been investigated using class II alloantisera and MLR assays (21, Davies et al. in preparation). These studies showed that the serological typing correlated well with DQ, DR RFLPs. Interestingly, some haplotypes which exhibited very similar, but not identical, RFLP patterns also shared class II allo-specificities. Furthermore, there was clear evidence that primary MLR reactions are controlled by genes in the DQ, DR subregion. No significant effect of the DO, DY subregion was revealed.

Acknowledgements. This work is supported by a grant from the Swedish Council for Forestry and Agricultural Research.

References

1. Amorena,B. and Stone,W.H. 1978. Serologically defined (SD) locus in cattle. Science 201:159-60.

2. Spooner,R.L., Leveziel,H., Grosclaude,F., Oliver,R.A., and Vaiman,M. 1978. Evidence for a possible major histocompatibility complex (BLA) in cattle. J.Immunogenet. 5:335-46.

3. Usinger,W.R., Curie-Cohen,M., and Stone,W.H. 1977. Lymphocyte-defined loci in cattle. Science 196:1017-18.

4. Usinger,W.R., Curie-Cohen,M., Benforado,K., Pringnitz,D., Rowe,R., Splitter,G.A., and Stone,W.H. 1981. The bovine major histocompatibility complex (BoLA): close linkage of the genes controlling serologically defined antigens and mixed lymphocyte reactivity. Immunogenetics 14:423-28.

5. Andersson,L. 1987. Genetic polymorphism of a bovine t-complex gene (TCP1). Linkage to major histocompatibility genes. J.Hered. In press.

6. Andersson,L. and Rask,L. 1987. Characterization of the MHC class II region in cattle. The number of DQ genes varies between haplotypes. Immunogenetics. In press.

7. Andersson,L., Böhme,J., Rask,L., and Peterson,P.A. 1986. Genomic hybridization of bovine major histocompatibility genes: 1. Extensive polymorphism of bovine DQα and DQβ genes. Anim.Genet. 17:95-112.

8. Andersson,L., Böhme,J., Peterson,P.A., and Rask,L. 1986. Genomic hybridization of bovine class II major histocompatibility genes: 2. Polymorphism of DR genes and linkage disequilibrium in the DQ-DR region. Anim.Genet. 17:295-304.

9. Andersson,L., Lundén,A., Sigurdardottir,S., Davies,C.J., and Rask,L. 1987. Linkage relationships in the bovine MHC region. High recombination frequency between class II subregions. Submitted for publication.

10. Sigurdardottir,S., Lundén,A., and Andersson,L.
     1987. Restriction fragment polymorphism of DQ and
     DR class II genes of the bovine MHC. In
     manuscript.

11. Barker,D., Schafer,M., and White,R. 1984.
     Restriction sites containing CpG show a higher
     frequency of polymorphism in human DNA. Cell
     36:131-38.

12. Tykocinski,M.L. and Max,E.C. 1984. CG
     dinucleotide clusters in MHC genes and in 5'
     demethylated genes. Nucleic Acids Res. 12:4385-
     96.

13. Silver,L.M. 1986. Mouse t haplotypes.
     Ann.Rev.Genet. 19:179-208.

14. Willison,K.R., Dudley,K., and Potter,J. 1986.
     Molecular cloning and sequence analysis of a
     haploid expressed gene encoding t complex
     polypeptide 1. Cell 44:727-38.

15. Leveziel,H. and Hines,H.C. 1984. Linkage in
     cattle between the major histocompatibility
     complex (BoLA) and the M blood group system.
     Génét.Sél.Evol. 16:405-16.

16. Bodmer,W.F., Trowsdale,J., Young,J., and
     Bodmer,J. 1986. Gene clusters and the evolution
     of the major histocompatibility system.
     Phil.Trans.R.Soc.Lond.B. 312:303-15.

17. Hardy,D.A., Bell,J.I., Long,E.O., Lindsten,T.,
     and McDevitt,H.O. 1986. Mapping of the class II
     region of the human major histocompatibility
     complex by pulsed-field electrophoresis. Nature
     323:453-55.

18. Steinmetz,M., Stephan,D., and Fischer-Lindahl,K.
     1986. Gene organization and recombination
     hotspots in the murine major histocompatibility
     complex. Cell 44:895-904.

19. Fisher,R.A. 1930. The Genetical Theory of Natural
     Selection. Oxford: Clarendon Press.

20. Germain,R.N., Bentley,D.M., and Quill,H. 1985.
     Influence of allelic polymorphism on the assembly
     and surface expression of class II MHC (Ia)
     molecules. Cell 43:233-42.

21. Davies,C.J. 1987. Immunogenetic characterization
     of the class II region of the bovine major
     histocompatibility complex. Ph.D. thesis, Cornell
     University, Ithaca, U.S.A.

Structure and Expression of Class I MHC Genes in the Miniature Swine

Dinah S. Singer, Rachel Ehrlich, Hana Golding, Leonardo Satz, Leslie Parent, and Stuart Rudikoff

The class I MHC gene family of the miniature swine consists of 7 members, 5 of which have been isolated and characterized with respect to structure and expression. DNA sequence analysis of these five genes reveals the existence of at least three sub-families. Four of the five genes are expressed in transfected L cells, although at different levels. Three are known to be expressed in vivo. One, PD15, is not expressed either in transfected L cells or in vivo, and may be a pseudogene.

Studies on the in vivo expression of the class I genes have focused on PD1, which encodes a major transplantation antigen, and PD6 which is the most divergent member of the family. The in vivo patterns of expression of both genes are generally similar: expression is highest in lymphoid tissues and lower in other tissues, such as kidney and liver. However, in the thymus, PD1 is expressed but PD6 is not. In contrast, in lymphoid populations, PD6 is preferentially expressed in T cells, whereas PD1 is preferentially expressed in B cells.

Molecular analyses of the regulatory elements governing the expression of PD1 have identified the transcriptional promoter and an interferon response element. The promoter is located between -38 and -220 bp upstream of translational initiation, whereas the interferon response element is located between -38 and -528 bp.

The class I genes of the major histocompatibility complex (MHC) comprise a family of homologous DNA sequences, some of which encode the heavy chain moiety of classical transplantation antigens found on the surface of all somatic cells. The major functions currently associated with the transplantation antigens are mediation of graft rejection and participation as restriction elements for antigen recognition (1-3). Class I molecules are expressed on all nucleated cells, with the exception of neurons and mature trophoblasts (4,5). However, the level of expression varies: the highest levels of class I antigens are found on lymphoid cells, while much lower levels occur in other somatic tissues. Further variation in the level of class I antigen expression can be caused by exogenous and endogenous factors, such as tumor necrosis factor, α/β-interferon or γ-interferon (6-11). The extent to which these varying levels of cell-surface antigen expression reflect differential expression of members of the family versus differential rates of expression of a few members is not known. To address this question, we have undertaken a detailed analysis of the structure, in vivo patterns of expression, and regulation of expression of the members of the class I MHC gene family of

Singer, Ehrlich, Golding, Satz, and Parent: Immunol. Branch, NIH, Bethesda, Md. Rudikoff: Lab. of Genet., NIH, Bethesda, Md.

the miniature swine (SLA). In this paper, we will summarize our current understanding of the structure and expression of this family.

   The SLA Class I Gene Family Contains Seven Members. In both mouse and man, the class I MHC gene families contain between 17 and 40 homologous sequences (12-15). To assess the size of the class I gene family in the miniature swine, genomic DNA was isolated and analyzed by Southern transfer procedures and hybridization with a class I specific DNA probe. The results of such an analysis, following digestion of the DNA with the restriction endonuclease Eco RI, are shown in Figure 1. A strikingly simple pattern of hybridization is observed, with only 5 major bands revealed.

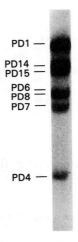

Figure 1. The genome of the miniature swine contains only 7 class I genes. Genomic DNA was digested with Eco RI, resolved on an agarose gel, blotted and hybridized with a probe derived from PD1.

   In order to further characterize the family, and its individual members, genomic recombinant DNA libraries, both bacteriophage and cosmid libraries, were constructed and screened for the presence of class I sequences. To date, 5 genes have been isolated. All of the genes isolated corresponded to hybridizing bands observed in the total genomic DNA digests. In repeated screenings of multiple libraries, no unexpected genes were isolated. From this and other studies (16), it appears that the class I family of the miniature swine is much smaller than that of any other species examined, consisting of only 7 members.

   To determine the structure and coding capacities of each of the genes, as well as their relationships to one another, their DNA sequences have been entirely determined (16,17). Four of the genes, PD1, PD14, PD6, and PD7 have the characteristic organization of a class I gene. That is, each consists of eight exons, which separately encode a leader domain, three extracytoplasmic domains, a transmembrane domain, and an

intracytoplasmic tail. All four genes contain open reading
frames in all exons, as well as legitimate splice sites. Thus,
at least four of the seven class I genes in the miniature swine
are capable of encoding class I antigens. The fifth sequence
analyzed, PD15, differs from the others in that there are no
sequences homologous to exons 5-8; the segment encoding the 5'
end of the gene has not yet been determined. Comparison of the
DNA sequences of these genes reveals the presence of at least
three sub-families (Table I). One sub-family consists of PD1,
PD14 and PD7; all three sequences are 80-85% homologous to one
another. Previous studies have demonstrated that PD1 and PD14
encode the major transplantation antigens of the miniature swine
(17,18). The product of PD7 remains to be identified. In
contrast to this relatively high homology among these three
genes, their homology to PD6 or PD15 is between 49 and 55%
(Table I). However, PD6 and PD15 are only 45% homologous to each
other and so define distinct families.

Table I. Relationships among the Class I MHC Genes of the
miniature swine

DNA SEQUENCE HOMOLOGY (%)[a]

Gene:	PD1	PD7	PD14	PD15	PD6
PD1	100	81	84	52	52
PD7	-	100	85	55	49
PD14	-	-	100	52	55
PD15	-	-	-	100	45

[a].DNA sequences comparisons are overall homologies, including
exons and introns.

The chromosomal organization of the SLA genes is not known
precisely. In situ hybridization studies have shown that all of
the class I genes are linked on chromosome 7 (19). The order of
the genes, and whether they are organized according to sub-
family is currently being determined by the techniques of
pulsed-field electrophoresis and chromosome walking using
overlapping cosmid clones. Preliminary results suggest that
there may be linkage of members of a sub-family. Thus, PD14 and
PD7, which belong to the same family have been isolated on a
single cosmid clone. PD6 which is the most divergent member of
the family, is also physically separated from the remaining
sequences.
Expression of the Class I MHC Genes.
        The antigen and RNA expression patterns of each of the
isolated genes are being assessed both in vivo and in
transfected L cells. The current status of this analysis is
summarized in Table II. Transfection of PD1, PD6, PD7 and PD14

into mouse L cells results in expression of SLA RNA (16-18).
However, cell surface expression of SLA antigens has only been
detected for PD1 and PD14. Studies are currently underway to
identify the products of PD6 and PD7.

Analysis of in vivo expression of these genes reveals
similar patterns: PD1, PD6, and PD14 have all been demonstrated
to be expressed in a variety of tissues in the miniature swine
(17,16, R. Ehrlich and D. Singer, in preparation). In contrast,
no in vivo expression of PD15 has been detected despite
extensive analysis of RNA samples from a variety of miniature
swine tissues (L. Parent and D. Singer, unpublished
observations). Among the genes which are expressed in vivo,
different patterns of expression are observed. Whereas both PD1
and PD6 are expressed at higher levels in lymphoid than in non-
lymphoid tissues, differences are apparent (Table III). Thus,
expression of PD1 is greater in thymus, heart and testis than in
kidney, whereas expression of PD6 is greater in kidney than in
thymus, heart or testis. The relative paucity of PD6 expression
in the thymus, relative to the other tissues is particularly

Table II. Isolation and Expression of Class I SLA Genes

GENE	ISOLATION	L CELLS		EXPRESSION IN VIVO
		ANTIGEN	RNA	
PD1	+	+	+	+
PD14	+	+	+	+
PD6	+	-	+	+
PD15	+	-	-	-
PD7	+	-	-/+	ND
PD4	-	ND	ND	ND
PD8	-	ND	ND	ND

striking in light of its preferential expression in T cells
(Table IV). Whereas PD1 expression is greater in B than in T
cells, PD6   expression is greater in T cells than in B cells.
From these analyses it is possible to conclude that individual
members of the SLA class I MHC gene family are differentially
regulated in vivo.

Identification and Mapping of Regulatory DNA Sequence Elements
in the 5' Flanking Region of PD1.

In order to establish the molecular mechanisms regulating the
in vivo patterns of expression of the class I SLA genes, we have
undertaken an extensive dissection of the 5' flanking regions of
these genes. Transfection of mouse L cells with the intact PD1
gene and its 5' flanking sequences results in the regulated cell
surface expression of PD1 antigens (10,21). In order to
functionally define the promoter, a series of deletion mutants
was constructed within the 5' end of PD1 (Figure 2).

Table III. Patterns of Expression of PD1 and PD6 in Different
           Tissues of the Miniature Swine.[a]

Tissue	PD1	PD6
Kidney	1	1
Heart	2.0	0.4
Testis	1.3	0
Liver	1.7	1.2
Lung	3.8	11.2
Lymph Node	5.2	18.8
Spleen	3.7	6.1
Thymus	1.8	0.2
PBL	11.4	ND

[a.] Levels of specific RNA were determined by S1 analysis using
DNA probes which had been demonstrated to be sequence
specific. Intensities of specific S1 protected bands were
determined by densitometry. RNA samples from the tissues were
all processed in parallel, using the same hybridizing probe
for each gene. The data presented are the average values of
two experiments using separate RNA preparations. Data have
been normalized to the intensity of the kidney specific bands
(absolute values of 0.29, 0.76 for PD1 and 0.25, 1.26 for
PD6).

Table IV. Relative Expression of PD1 and PD6 in T Cells and B
          cells.[a]

Gene	Relative RNA levels (T cell/B cell)
PD1	0.36
PD6	1.4

[a.] Lymphocyte populations were purified as described (16).
Levels of specific RNA were determined as in Table III.

The 5' termini of the mutants were located either at a Hind III
site at -1121 (pH series) or at an Nde I site at -528 (pN
series). A nested set of deletions (spanning nucleotides +15 to
-236) was generated by Bal 31 exonuclease digestion from a
unique Sac I site located within intron 1. The precise locations
of the deletion end-points were determined by DNA sequence
analysis, and are indicated in Figure 2. The deletion mutants
were cloned into the promoter assay vector, pSV0CAT, which lacks
eukaryotic promoters or enhancers, and tested for their ability
to promote the synthesis of chloramphenicol acetyl transferase
(CAT) following transfection into mouse L cells. Whereas both
pH(+15) and pH(-38) are able to promote the synthesis of CAT

enzyme, pH(-220) was unable to do so (Figure 3). Thus, DNA
sequences between -38 bp and -220 bp are required for promoter
activity. Since both pN(+15) and pN(-38) are able to promote
synthesis of CAT, DNA sequences between -528 bp and -1121 bp are
not necessary for promoter activity. The ability of the PD1 DNA
segment to direct the synthesis of CAT is orientation dependent,
as evidenced by the observation that insertion of the Hind
II/Sac I PD1 segment in the opposite orientation [p(+255)H] did
not promote CAT activity. S1 nuclease analysis of RNA derived
from L cells stably transfected with pH(-38) revealed only a
single initiation site, mapping near the PD1/CAT junction (data
not shown). These results demonstrate that DNA sequence elements
necessary and sufficient for promoter actiivty are located
between positions -38 and -528 bp. DNA sequencing of this region
(data not shown) reveals the presence of the elements ACCC,
CCAAT and TCTAA, which have been associated with promoter
activity in other systems, suggesting that these elements
contribute to the class I promoter.

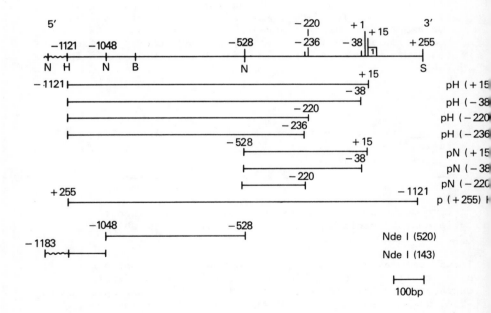

Figure 2. Map of DNA sequence of PD1 5' flanking region. DNA
deletion fragments containing PD1 5' flanking sequence, indicated
by solid line, were inserted into the Hind III site of pSV0.
N indicates Nde I; H, Hind III; B, Bgl II; S, Sac I.

Treatment of PD1-transfected mouse L cells with α/β-interferon results in increased expression of both endogenous H-2 and exogenous SLA, both of which range between 1.5 and 2-fold (10). The effect of α/β-interferon on L cell transfectants containing the various PD1-promoter CAT constructs was assessed in order to determine whether the interferon responsive element(s) mapped to the 5' region of the PD1 gene. Interferon treatment of L cells tranfected with either pH(-38) or pH(+15) resulted in increased levels of intracellular CAT activity (Figure 4). The extent of this increase, as determined by densitometric analysis ranged between 1.5-2 fold in different experiments. The interferon responsive element is promoter dependent, since interferon does

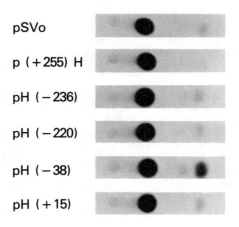

pSVo

p (+255) H

pH (-236)

pH (-220)

pH (-38)

pH (+15)

Figure 3. Mapping of PD1 promoter. Mouse L cells were transfected with the indicated DNA constructs. 48 hours later, cells were harvested and extracts assayed for CAT activity.

	IFN		Ratio of CAT Activity (+IFN/−IFN)
pH (−38)	+ −		1.51
pH (+15)	+ −		1.4
p (+255) H	+ −		0
pH (−220)	+ −		0
pSV1	+ −		0.97
pN (−38)	+ −		1.61
pN (+15)	+ −		1.44

Figure 4. Mouse L cells were stably transfected with the indicated DNA constructs and cultured in the presence or absence of α/β interferon for 24 hours. Cells were harvested and extracts assayed for CAT activity. The ratios are the average of two experiments.

not induce de novo CAT activity in L cells transfected with either pH(-220) or p(+255)H (Figure 4). Interferon also has no effect on the level of CAT activity generated by the SV40 promoter in L cells transfected with pSV1CAT. Thus, an interferon responsive element(s) is present within the 5' flanking region of PD1 and can account for the observed response of the intact gene. To further map the location of the interferon responsive element, the responses of L cell transfectants generated from pN(-38) and pN(+15), which have 5' end truncations (Figure 2), were analyzed. Both cell lines were fully capable of responding to interferon to the same extent as those containing the parental constructs (Figure 4). Thus, the interferon responsive element(s) is located within 500 bp of initiation of transcription. An interferon consensus sequence of 29 bp has been reported for a number of genes, including an HLA class I gene (21). The PD1 gene, between -209 and -180 bp, has a sequence with 69% homology to this consensus sequence (R. Ehrlich, J. Maguire, and D. Singer, submitted). It remains to be established whether this particular DNA sequence of PD1 constitutes the interferon response element for the SLA gene and whether its function is dependent on the existence of other 5' flanking sequences.

Conclusions.

Of the seven class I SLA genes in the genome of the miniature swine, five have been isolated and are being characterized. DNA sequence analysis has revealed the existence of at least three sub-families, defined by the higher homology within the sub-family than between members of different sub-families. Analysis of in vivo patterns of expression of the class I genes suggests molecular mechanisms for both coordinate and differential regulation of expression. Thus, although both PD1 and PD6 show overall similarities in their patterns of expression, striking differences are seen in the thymus and lymphocytes. PD1, but not PD6, is expressed in the thymus. In lymphocytes, PD6 is preferentially expressed in T cells and PD1 in B cells. Molecular analysis of the 5' flanking DNA segment of PD1 has allowed the identification of the transcriptional promoter, as well as an interferon responsive element. Future studies will focus on the identification of other regulatory elements contained within the PD1 segment, as well as the regulatory elements associated with PD6. Comparison of the regulatory elements of PD1 and PD6 should yield insights into the molecular mechanisms regulating their patterns of tissue expression.

REFERENCES

1. Klein, J. 1979. The major histocompatibility complex of the mouse. Science. 203:516:521.
2. Klein, J. 1975. Biology of the mouse histocompatibility complex.
3. Klein, J. 1977. Major Histocompatibility Complex. eds. Gotze, E.
4. Faulk, W.D., A.R. Sanderson, and A. Temple. 1977. Distribution of MHC antigens in human placental chorionic villi. Transplant. Proc. 9:1379-1384.
5. Lampson, L.A., C.A. Fisher, and J.P. Whelan. 1983. Striking paucity of HLA-ABC and $beta_2$-microglobulin on human neuroblastoma cell lines. J. Immunol. 130:2471-2478.
6. Burrone, O.H., and C. Milstein. 1982. Control of HLA-A, B, C synthesis and expression in interferon treated cells. EMBO Journal. 1:345-349.
7. Collins, T., L.A. Lapierre, W. Fiers, J.L. Strominger, and J.S. Pober. 1986. Recombinant human tumor necrosis factor increases mRNA levels and surface expression of HLA-A,B antigens in vascular endothelial cells and dermal fibroblasts in vitro. Proc. Natl. Acad. Sciences (USA). 83:446-450.
8. Imai, K., M.A. Pellegrino, A.K. Ng, and S. Ferron. 1981. Role of antigen density in immune lysis of interferon-treated human lymphoid cells. Scand. J. Immunol. 14:529-535.
9. Lindhal, P., P. Leary, and I. Gresser. 1973. Enhancement by interferon of the expression of histocompatibility antigens of mouse lymphoid cells. Eur. J. Immunol. 4:779-784.
10. Satz, M., and D.S. Singer. 1984. Effect of mouse interferon on the expression of the porcine MHC gene introduced into mouse L-cells. J. Immunol. 132:496-501.
11. Wallach, D.M., M. Fellous, and M. Revel. 1982. Preferential effect of gamma interferon on the synthesis of HLA antigens and their mRNA's in human cells. Nature. 299:833-836.
12. Cohen, D., P. Paul, M. Font, O. Cohen, B. Sayagh, A. Marcadet, M. Busson, G. Majory, H. Cann, and J. Dausset. 1983. Analysis of HLA class I genes with restriction endonuclease fragments. Implications for polymorphism of the human major histocompatibility complex. Proc. Natl. Acad. Science (USA). 80:6289-6292.
13. Orr, H., R. Bach, H. Ploegh, J.L. Strominger, P. Kavathas, and R. DeMars. 1982. Use of HLA loss mutants to analyse the structure of the human MHC. Nature. 296:454-456.
14. Steinmetz, M., A. Winoto, K. Minard, and L. Hood. 1982. Clustering of genes encoding mouse transplantation antigens. Cell. 28:489-498.
15. Weiss, E.H., L. Golden, K. Fahrner, A. Mellor, H. Devlin, H. Tiddens, H. Bud, and R.A. Flavell. 1984. Organization and evolution of the class I gene family in the MHC of the C57BL/10 mouse. Nature. 310:650-655.

16. Ehrlich, R., R. Lifshitz, M. Pescovitz, S. Rudikoff, and
    D.S. Singer. 1987. Tissue specific expression and structure
    of a divergent member of a class I MHC gene family. J.
    Immunol. 139:593-602.
17. Satz, M., L.C. Wang, D.S. Singer, and S. Rudikoff. 1985.
    Structure and expression of two porcine genomic clones
    encoding class I MHC antigens. J. Immunol. 135:2167-2175.
18. Singer, D.S., M. Camerini-Otero, M. Satz, B. Osborne, D.
    Sachs, and S. Rudikoff. 1982. Characterization of a porcine
    genomic clone encoding a major transplantation antigen;
    expression in mouse L-cells. Proc. Natl. Acad. Sciences
    (USA). 79:1403-1407.
19. Rabin, M., R. Fries, D.S. Singer, and F. Ruddle. 1985.
    Assignment of the porcine major histocompatibility complex to
    chromosome 7 by in situ hybridization. Cytogenet. Cell Genet.
    39:206-209.
20. Satz, M. L., and D. S. Singer. 1983. Differential expression
    of porcine major histocompatibility DNA sequences introduced
    into mouse L cells. Molec. Cell. Biol. 3:2006-2016.
21. Friedman, R., and G. Stark. 1985. Alpha interferon induces
    transcription of HLA and metallothionein genes which have
    homologous upstream sequences. Nature 314:637-639.

Genetic Organization of the SLA Complex

P. Chardon, Cl. Geffrotin, and M. Vaiman

Knowledge concerning the overall organization of chromosome 7 in swine, especially the region comprising SLA, the Major Histocompatibility Complex, has greatly progressed in recent years, thanks to direct gene mapping, the RFLP technique and by gene cloning. Hybridization of class I probes on Eco-Rl digests of swine genomic DNA revealed about 10 bands in individual homozygotes for the SLA complex. This is markedly less than in the other livestock species investigated. Some of the swine class I bands were found to correlate with certain serologically-defined class I specificities. On the basis of the results obtained with HLA class II probes, the SLA class II region appears to contain up to 10 beta DR-related sequences but fewer beta DQ genes and possibly no more than one or two DR and DQ alpha genes. Restriction site variability was obvious for all these genes. Studies of several SLA recombinants in selected families showed that all the class II genes are tightly clustered inside the SLA-D-MLR region. The SLA class I and class II DNA sequences belong to two distinct regions, and no specific sequences from either class are interspersed with sequences of the other. The C4 region was mapped inside the SLA complex by RFLP but the presence of one or several C4 genes could not be ascertained. Analysis of cosmid clones from swine genomic DNA revealed that the C4 and 21 hydroxylase genes are tightly linked.

THE HISTORY of the pig major histocompatibility complex (MHC) covers a rather long period as it was already characterized by 1970. A relationship was first established between acute graft rejection and a set of membrane antigens expressed by peripheral blood lymphocytes. These antigens were found to be controlled by a cluster of genes which had a mendelian inheritance and in fact constituted the MHC of the pig, also referred to as the swine lymphocyte antigen complex (SLA) (35). Since the MHC was first described, knowledge about this complex in the pig has steadily grown, thanks to serological, histochemical and biochemical analyses. In addition, the mixed lymphocyte reaction (MLR) has revealed another facet of this complex (3,34).

The SLA complex comprises two main regions (figure 1) : one of them is homologous to the human class I and controls the transplantation antigens (the so-called class I molecules) directly involved in graft rejection and allogeneic restriction. Three series of class I SLA loci have been described in the pig: of these, the A and B loci have been identified thanks to the discovery of genetic recombinants, and the existence of

Chardon: INRA Laboratoire de Radiobiologie Appliquée 78350 Jouy-en-Josas, France. Geffrotin and Vaiman: CEA-IPSN-DPS-SPE Laboratoire de Radiobiologie Appliquée 91191 Gif sur Yvette, France.

the C locus has been inferred from the results of biochemical
and serological experiments (36). Class I pig transplantation
antigens exhibit the characteristic dimeric structure of class
I molecules and comprise a beta 2 microglobulin non-covalently
associated with a 43 KD glycosylated polypeptide (6,26). The
latter is highly polymorphic and about 40 different specificities are known today among the various breeds of pig.

The second chromosomal region - the D region - is homologous to the human class II region and controls the MLR. From a
biochemical point of view, this region codes for two series of
class II molecules consisting of two glycosylated polypeptides
of 33 and 29 KD respectively (7,27). So far, we have collected
12 SLA homozygous typing cells, constituting distinct D alleles. The class I and class II regions are about 0.4 centimorgans apart.

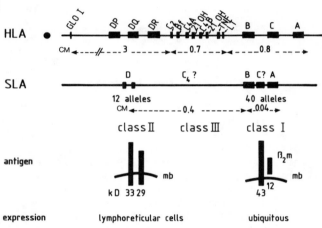

Figure 1 : Comparison of the genetic maps of the HLA and SLA
complex as defined by serological, biochemical and mixed
lymphocyte reaction studies. The analogous regions of both
MHCs are lined up in order to facilitate the comparison, but
in fact the relative position of each SLA region has not yet
been determined.
KD : kilodalton ; CM : centimorgan

Besides the class I and class II genes directly involved
in immune responses, several other unrelated families of genes
appear to be non-randomly linked to the mammal MHC region. For
instance, in man and mouse, what is termed the class III
region comprises genes coding for two related C2 and B factor
genes and a third C4 gene, all involved in complement pathway
activation (28).   Close to C4 there is a gene coding for the
21 hydroxylase enzyme (21-OH), a cytochrome molecule which

belongs to the P450 family and is active in the metabolism of the steroid hormones in the adrenal cortex (37). As shown in the schematic pathway drawn in figure 2, 21-OH converts 17 hydroxyprogesterone into deoxycortisol, and progesterone into deoxycorticosterone, leading to cortisol or aldosterone production. Since mutations or deletions in the coding 21-OH gene, which are quite frequent in humans, can modify this gene's activity, the steroid pathway may be diverted and drastically reduce adrenal hormone synthesis while enhancing that of testosterone.

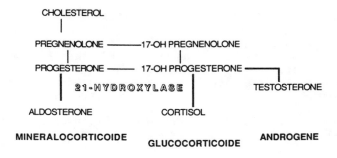

Figure 2 : Effect of 21-hydroxylase on metabolic pathway of steroid hormones in the adrenal cortex.

Recently, structural genes for the tumor necrosis factor and lymphotoxin, which play a crucial role in defense against tumor growth, have been located in the class III region (18).

In the pig, the SLA class III region is as yet ill defined. We previously showed that the SLA complex affects complement-dependent hemolytic activity, presumably by means of class III molecules. We subsequently suggested that in pig the C4 gene is located inside the SLA complex (22). Because of the potential interest in genes like 21-OH in pig, we attempted to establish whether such genes are also located inside the SLA region. Until now, porcine steroid 21-OH has only been studied at the protein level. YUAN and coll. (39) isolated, from porcine adrenocortical microsomes, a 54 KD molecule with two NH-2 terminal sequences, one of which lacked the NH-2 terminal methionine. This molecule was extremely hydrophobic and hardly displayed any homology, either to the porcine 17 alpha hydroxylase C-17,20 lyase isolated from neonatal testes, or to rabbit and rat liver microsomal P450 cytochromes. Comparison of the incomplete porcine 21-OH amino acid sequence with the sequences of human and bovine 21-OH enzymes reveals a good homology between them (2). However, nothing was known about pig 21-OH at the molecular level, and this review includes our preliminary results for 21-OH genes.

A large number of human and murine DNA probes corresponding to different MHC genes have been cloned during recent years. Because these genes have been remarkably well preserved during evolution the related probes can be used directly at the DNA level for detailed investigation of the organization and polymorphism of SLA genes. The first results obtained using such probes concern the mapping of the SLA complex.

CHROMOSOMAL ASSIGNMENT OF THE SLA COMPLEX

We performed direct in situ hybridization on chromosomes in spread metaphases. Using the HLA B7 class I probe (31) which recognizes homologous sequences in pig genomic DNA, we obtained a specific signal in the Q2-1 region of chromosome 7 (17)(figure 3). Subsequently, a more precise location was proposed by RABIN and coll. (29), ECHARD and coll. (13) and FRIES and coll.(16). The SLA complex was eventually located in the P1-1 region.

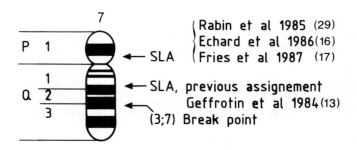

Figure 3 : Mapping of the SLA complex. In situ hybridization on spread metaphases were performed using the HLA class I probe (13,16) or the specific SLA class I probe (17,29).

Nevertheless, serological results favored the initial Q2-1 location (Ch. RENARD personal communication). In several families of pigs in which a translocated 3-7 P(1:3) Q(2:1) chromosome was present we only observed a few recombinants between the SLA antigens and the second marker constituted by the break point. The latter is located distally on the long arm of chromosome 7. In all, only 5 recombinations were observed out of 68 informative haplotypes (figure 4). The lod score analysis gave an estimated recombination rate of theta = 8%.

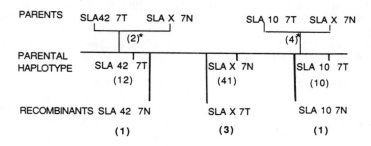

Figure 4 : Segregation of SLA specificities in families
bearing the (3-7) translocated chromosome.
N   : normal chromosome 7
7T   : 3-7 P(1:3) Q(2:1) translocated chromosome
( )   : number of piglets
( )* : number of families

These observations bear out our initial assignment of the
SLA region to the long arm. However, the existence of a cross-
over inhibitory mechanism due to the translocation, which   may
artificially lower lod score values, cannot be ruled out.

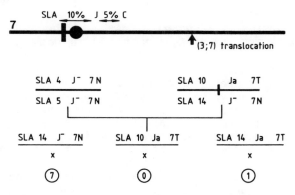

Figure 5 : Linkage between SLA complex and the J blood group
system. Segregation of SLA specificities in a family where the
sow carried a translocated chromosome 7. The piglet presenting
the SLA 14-Ja specificities on the translocated chromosome was
recombinant.
7T   : 3-7 P(1:3) Q(2:1) translocated chromosome.
7N   : normal chromosome 7.
( )   : number of piglets.

One of the few recombinants observed allowed us to locate
the J blood group locus between the SLA region and the break

point. Since HRUBAN and Coll.(21) reported several years ago that the SLA complex was 10 centimorgans away from the J blood group and that this group was 5 centimorgans from the C blood group system, the three markers can be clearly ordered as described in figure 5.

Somatic hybrids between pig and hamster cells have been used to test for synteny between SLA and certain isoenzyme loci. A synteny between nucleoside phosphorylase (NP) and mannose phosphate isomerase (MPi) has been described by DOLF (11) and assigned to chromosome 7. Pyruvate kinase (PKM2) was also found to be syntenic with NP and MPi (12). The NP locus was recently located in the Q2 region of chromosome 7 by YERLE (personal communication) using in situ hybridization with a radiolabeled NP probe.

Synteny was excluded for superoxide dismutase 2 and no informative results were obtained for malic enzyme, phosphoglucomutase 3 or glyoxalase 1 (GLO 1). All of these isoenzymes belong to the HLA linkage group and are also syntenic in the cat (40). Nevertheless LIE and coll. (25) demonstrated a link between the GLO 1 locus and the SLA complex by showing quantitative differences in GLO 1 activity as a function of SLA haplotypes. This finding agrees with the fact that GLO 1 is always found close to mammal MHC.

EXPLORATION OF THE SLA CLASS I REGION AT THE MOLECULAR LEVEL.

Using the Southern blot technique (32) and an HLA specific class I cDNA probe, SINGER and coll. demonstrated the possibility of analyzing the pig MHC complex at the molecular level (30). The probe hybridized with numerous bands of pig DNA digested with EcoRI or Bam HI endonucleases. A specific banding pattern was obtained for each of the three miniature pig haplotypes, although a certain number of bands were common to them all. The same authors successively isolated three clones (14) containing functional SLA class-I genes from a miniature swine genomic library prepared from an SLA d homozygote. The transcription of one of these genes appeared to be regulated in a particular fashion. A porcine SLA class I gene was successfully introduced into the genome of a C57BL/10 mouse (15), where it was found to behave like a single mendelian locus and to function as a transplantation antigen.

Southern blotting and molecular cross-hybridization have also been performed in unrelated pigs (8) and in SLA-informative families (9) from Large White or Landrace breeds, using the HLA class I probe specified above. The results confirmed the considerable molecular polymorphism found in miniature pigs, as few bands were common to any of the 13 distinct haplotypes in the commercial breeds. It was interesting to observe that one group of SLA A15 C1 B18 serologically indistinguishable unrelated homozygotes clearly split into two groups, showing that further polymorphism may be found at the DNA level.

In families where the parents expressed distinct SLA haplotypes, an average of 15 to 16 bands was obtained after Eco-RI digestion and hybridization with the HLA class I probe. Polymorphic restriction fragments segregated without exception, in accordance with the serological typing.

Conservation of MHC class I region concerns not only MHC organization but also gene structure. Thus, SLA class I genes, like human genes, consist of eight exons, of which exon 2 displayed the greatest heterogeneity (30).

In conclusion, there are more SLA class I genes at the DNA level than are actually expressed. It is not known which of the bands corresponds to SLA functional genes, nor whether the remainder represent pseudogenes or pig genes related to the mouse Qa-Tla family. As already stressed by EHRLICH and coll. (14), there is a strikingly small number of SLA class I sequences. It appears that no more than 6 to 8 class I genes per haploid genome exist in the pig, a figure two to three times lower than for any of the other mammals so far analyzed, including man.

MOLECULAR ANALYSIS OF THE SLA CLASS II REGION.

Various labeled HLA class II probes specific for HLA-DQ (23,1) and DR genes (20,24) coding for heavy and light chains were serially hybridized with Eco-RI or Bam HI digested genomic DNA from pigs of different origins (8,9). The results can be summarized as follows: a) after Eco-RI cleavage of DNA from SLA heterozygotes, the HLA-DR beta probe revealed the existence of about sixteen bands i.e. 6 to 8 genes per haplotype. Many of these bands were polymorphic and when observed in families, always followed the haplotype segregation as revealed by MLR tests. b) The number of bands obtained by hybridization with a human DQ beta probe never exceeded five or six for a given individual. Usually, one or two intense bands were accompanied by several faint ones, and some of the DQ beta bands appeared to cross-react with DR beta bands. c) The SLA DQ-like and SLA DR-like heavy chain gene families, appeared to be even smaller than the light-chain gene families as no more than 2 bands were observed in any individual. However, with appropriate restriction enzymes, polymorphic fragments were generated. d) Preliminary tests with a specific DP beta probe yielded no clear hybridizing band, suggesting that no sequence closely resembling DP exists in the pig genome. Analysis of several SLA recombinants with all four class II probes confirmed that all the class II genes were clustered inside the SLA region originally defined by MLR. Furthermore, no alteration in any of the class II bands was observed, which was consistent with the results of the MLR tests.

The conclusion is that the SLA class II region probably contains a large number of DR light chain coding genes and probably also several DQ light chain genes. However, this region apparently includes very few SLA genes coding for DR and DQ heavy chains.

SLA CLASS III REGION.

Pig hemolytic complement activity was found to be influenced by the SLA complex. More direct evidence for the presence of a complement gene within the SLA region was obtained by Southern blot hybridization using a human cDNA C4 probe of 300 base pairs (5). Hybridization to Eco-RI digested genomic DNA from a SLA-informative family revealed a C4 polymorphic band which cosegregated with one SLA haplotype (22). Similar hybridization experiments on several of the above-mentioned SLA recombinants and their families did not enable more precise mapping of the C4 gene(s) within the SLA complex, because of the absence of polymorphic bands.

Further investigations of the SLA class III region were performed using human probes (4,33) specific for C2, B or 21-OH genes. Although all these probes hybridized with swine DNA, these genes could not be assigned because of the absence of variability in the restriction sites in the range of enzymes used. Since we considered that the class III region is of potential importance for performance traits, we decided to begin exploring the class III region in detail.

The gene coding for the 21-OH enzyme was first mapped by flow sorting chromosomes and spot hybridization. Pig flow karyotypes from both sexes display 13 peaks for the 18 autosomal pairs and the two sexual chromosomes. A modification of the flow karyotype was readily detectable for the (3,7) translocation (19).

A certain number of chromosomes were assigned to different peaks and sorted. Hybridizations using heterologous probes after appropriate treatment and denaturation confirmed the mapping of SLA on chromosome 7 and suggested that the 21-OH gene was also present on this chromosome.

A genomic DNA library was then constructed and we tried to isolate and characterize the C4 and 21OH genes by picking out the related sequences using human and murine probes. Although this work is still preliminary, it has already supplied a certain amount of new information.

The library was built in the Lorist B vector, a new cosmid constructed by Cross and Little (10). This cosmid contains the kanamicin resistance gene and the lambda origin of replication. It also includes the SP-6 and T7 RNA polymerase promoter sequences that are orientated towards and adjacent to the Bam HI cloning site. One of the original features of the recombinant Lorist B cosmids consists of an in-vivo packaging procedure that produces molecules with normal cohesive ends allowing the use of the cos mapping technic.

The genomic DNA was prepared from an SLA H1 homozygous pig and partially digested by Sau 3A endonuclease, in order to obtain inserts of about 40.000 base pairs. From this library of about 350000 recombinants, three positive cosmids recognized by the human C4 cDNA probe of 300 bp (5), two recognized by the murine 21-OH probe (33) and one recognized by both probes were selected.

We first focused our attention on the latter. After partial digestion with Eco-RI and Bam HI endonucleases, cos mapping gave the preliminary restriction map displayed in figure 6. Both probes recognized fragments of about 4.9 kilobases after Bam HI, and 9 kilobases after Eco-RI digestion. Those are the sizes expected from the pattern obtained after digestion of pig genomic DNA using the same enzymes. The results of double digestion with these enzymes were also in agreement for both insert and genomic DNA. The estimated distance between the C4 and 21-OH genes was about 4 kilobases, indicating that in pig, these genes are located close together within a DNA segment defined as the SLA class III region (figure 6). However, since reshuffling is not uncommon, especially in large inserts, further confirmation is needed. Studies are in progress using a complete human cDNA C4 probe instead of the above mentioned probe. Thus the complete cDNA probe revealed five bands when tested on Bam HI digested porcine genomic DNA, and therefore is more adequate to assign the various C4 gene fragments in the insert.

Cos mapping of other positive overlapping clones is now in progress. These clones apparently belong to the same cluster which spanned about 80 kb. This cluster seems to contain only one C4 and one 21OH gene. We are therefore now screening for new clones in the genomic library with 3' or 5' end insert sequences, in a search for other overlapping clones and the still hypothetical second C4 and 21-OH genes.

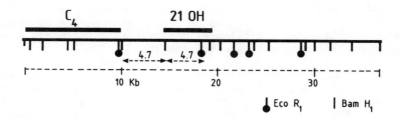

Figure 6 : Preliminary restriction map (cos mapping) of the cosmid positive with both C4 and 21-OH probes.

CONCLUSION

The overall results available for class I and class II genes clearly show the remarkable homology of the SLA complex with other MHC regions, particularly HLA and H-2, the best known MHC models (figure 7). The organization of the class I gene shown exhibits MHC conservation at a different level (30).

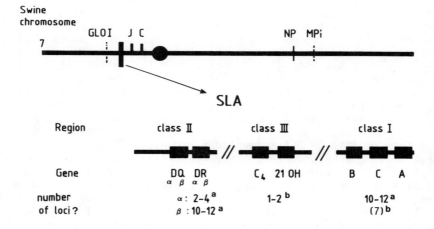

Figure 7 : Genetic organization of the SLA complex and its linkage group.
Glyoxalase 1 (GLO1) ; Nucleoside phosphorylase (NP) ; Mannose phosphate isomerase (MPi) ; 21-hydroxylase (21-OH) ; Blood group systems (J,C)
Hypothetical number of loci from : (a) RFLP studies
(b) cloning studies.

Nevertheless, some differences appear to exist. For instance there are only 6-7 class I sequences in pig, which is clearly fewer than in other mammal species including farm animals (14). The significance of this difference is not yet clear. On the other hand, the number of potential class II sequences comprising 10-12 genes for the beta DR-DQ-like chain and 2-4 genes for the alpha DR-DQ-like chain corresponds to the numbers found in other species.

Similarly, the class III region appears to contain C4 and 21-OH genes too. We do not yet know whether these genes are duplicated, as usually occurs in man and mouse. In these species, only one gene is in fact active and the other often seems to be a pseudogene (33,37). Further, duplication of C4 and 21-OH sequences in the mouse considerably altered the mechanism controlling these genes (33).

Taken together, the above observations concerning man and mouse constitute important issues with respect to the possible role of the homologous genes in pigs in determining physiological and performance traits. There is increasing evidence that the SLA region, like the H-2 region in mouse, is associated with various physiological pathways affecting zootechnical performances to a surprisingly large extent. For instance, we have already demonstrated that particular SLA haplotypes are correlated with various production traits such as the growth rate and carcass fatness, or even with reproduction traits like litter size, the ovulation rate, weight at birth or even piglet mortality. We might therefore be on the brink of a real breakthrough regarding the use of available knowledge concerning the SLA region in selection programs.

As mentioned above, physiologically important molecules, namely tumor necrosis factor and lymphotoxin, were recently shown to be controlled by genes inside the MHC region in man and mouse (18). It will be important to see whether these genes are also linked to the MHC region of other mammals, particularly livestock. In cattle for instance, a synteny between BoLA and 21-OH was recently described (38) and it will therefore be of interest to ascertain whether or not tumor necrosis factor and lymphotoxin genes are located inside the MHC region. Little is known about cytokines in domestic species, although these molecules might be partly responsible for important clinical and pathological symptoms.

In conclusion, the SLA region is progressively becoming the best known genomic region in the pig with more than 20 genes already characterized, and many more no doubt remain to be discovered. Accurate knowledge of this important region might radically affect future breeding and selection programs in pig species.

ACKNOWLEDGEMENTS

The contributions from R. Feil and S. Leger to this work were greatly appreciated. The skill of I. Chifflet in preparing the manuscript is acknowledged.

REFERENCES

1.   Auffray, C., Lillie, J.W., Arnot, D., Grossberger, D., Kappes, D. and Strominger J.L. 1984. Isotypic and allotypic variation of human class II histocompatibility antigen a-chain genes. Nature 308, 327-333.

2.   Bienkowski M.J., Haniu, M., Nakajin, S., Shinoda, M., Yanagibashi K., Hall P.F., and Shively, J.E. 1984. Peptide alignment of the porcine 21-hydroxylase cytochrome P-450 using a cDNA sequence of the corresponding bovine enzyme. Biochemical and Biophysical Research Communications 125, 734-740.

3.   Binns R.M. 1967. Bone marrow and lymphoid cell injection of the pig foetus resulting in transplantation tolerance or immunity, and immunoglobulin production. Nature, 214, 179-180.

4.   Campbell, R.D., and Porter, R.R. 1983. Molecular cloning and characterization of the gene coding for human complement protein factor B. Proceedings of the National Academy of Science (U.S.A.) 80, 4464-4468.

5.   Carroll, M.C., Campbell, R.D., and Porter, R.R. 1985. Mapping of steroid 21-hydroxylase genes adjacent to complement component C4 genes in HLA, the major histocompatibility complex in man. Proceedings of the National Academy of Science (U.S.A.) 82,521-525.

6.   Chardon, P., Vaiman, M., Renard, Ch., and Arnoux, B. 1978. Pig histocompatibility antigens and beta 2-microglobulin. Transplantation 26,107-112.

7.   Chardon, P., Renard, Ch., and Vaiman, M. 1981. Characterization of class II histocompatibility antigens in pigs. Anim. Blood Grps. and Biochem. Genet. 12, 59-65.

8.   Chardon, P., Vaiman, M., Kirszenbaum, M., Geffrotin, Cl., Renard, Ch. and Cohen, D. 1985. Restriction fragment length polymorphism of the major histocompatibility complex of the pig. Immunogenetics 21,161-171.

9. Chardon, P., Renard, Ch., Kirszenbaum, M., Geffrotin, Cl., Cohen, D. and Vaiman, M. 1985. Molecular genetic analyses of the major histocompatibility complex in pig families and recombinants. J. of Immunol. 12, 139-149.

10. Cross, S.H., Little, P.F.R. 1986. A cosmid vector for systematic chromosome walking. Gene 42,9-22.

11. Dolf, G.J., Stranzinger, G. 1986. Pig gene mapping : assignment of the genes for mannosephosphate isomerase (MPI) and nucleoside phosphorylase (NP) to chromosome no.7. Genet. Sel. Evol. 18, 375-384

12. Echard, E., Gellin, J. and Gillois, M. 1984. Localisation des gènes MPI, PKM2, NP sur le chromosome 3 du porc (Sus scrofa L.) et analyse cytogénétique d'une lignée de hamster chinois issue de la DON (wg3h). Genet. Sel. Evol. 16,261-270.

13. Echard, G., Yerle, N., Gellin, J., Dallens M. and Gillois, M. 1986. Assignment of the major histocompatibility complex to the q1.2 - p1.4 region of chromosome 7 in the pig (Sus scrofa domestica L.) by in situ hybridization. Cytogenet. Cell Genet. 41,126-128.

14. Ehrlich, R., Lifshitz, R., Pescovitz, M.D., Rudikoff, S. and Singer, D.S. 1987. Tissue-specific expression and structure of a divergent member of a class I MHC gene family. J. of Immunol. 139,593-602.

15. Frels, W.I., Bluestone, J.A., Hodes, R.J., Capecchi, M.R. and Singer, D.S. 1985. Expression of a microinjected porcine class I major histocompatibility complex gene in transgenic mice. Science 228,577-580.

16. Fries, R., Hedlger, R., Ansari, HA., Hetzel, D.J.S. and Stranzinger, G. 1987. Chromosomal assignment of the major histocompatibility complex in swine, cattle and horse by in situ hybridization. 9th human gene mapping. Paris, France.

17. Geffrotin, Cl, Popescu, C.P., Cribiu, E.P., Boscher, J., Renard, CH., Chardon, P. and Vaiman, M. 1984. Assignment of MHC in swine to chromosome 7 by in situ hybridization and serological typing. Annales de génétique 27,213-219.

18. Goeddel, D.V., Aggarwal, B.B., Gray, P.W., Leung, D.W, Nedwin, G.E., Palladino, M.A., Patton, J.S., Pennica, D., Shepard, H.M., Sugarman, B.J., and Wong, G.H.W. 1986. Tumor Necrosis Factors ; Gene Structure and Biological Activities. Cold Spring Harbor Symposia on Quantitative

Biology 51,597-609.

19. Grunwald, D., Geffrotin, Cl., Chardon, P., Frelat, G., and Vaiman, M. 1986. Swine chromosomes : Flow sorting and spot blot hybridization. Cytometry 7,582-588.

20. Gustafsson, K., Wiman, K., Emmoth, E., Larhammar, D., Bohme, J., Hyldig-Nielsen, J., Ronne, H., Peterson, P.A. and Rask, L. 1984. Mutations and selection in the generation of class II histocompatibility antigen polymorphism. The EMBO Journal 3,1655-1662.

21. Hruban, V., Simon, M., Hradecky, J. and Jilek, F. 1976. Linkage of the pig main histocompatibility complex and J. blood group system. Tissue Antigens 7,267-271.

22. Kirszenbaum, M., Renard, Ch., Geffrotin, Cl., Chardon, P., and Vaiman, M. 1985. Evidence for mapping pig C4 gene(s) within the pig major histocompatibility complex (SLA). Anim. Blood Grps. and Biochem. Genet. 16,65-68.

23. Larhammar, D., Schenning, L., Gustafsson, K., Wiman, K., Claesson, L., Rask, L. and Peterson P.A. 1982. Complete amino acid sequence of an HLA-DR antigen-like beta-chain as predicated from the nucleotide sequence : similarities with immunoglobulins and HLA-A,-B and -C antigens. Proceedings of the National Academy of Science (USA) 79,3687-3691.

24. Larhammar, D., Gustafsson, K., Claesson, L., Bill, P., Wiman, K., Schenning, L., Sundelin, J., Widmark, E., Peterson, P.A., and Rask, L. 1982. Alpha Chain of HLA-DR Transplantation Antigens is a Member of the Same Protein Superfamily as the Immunoglobulins. Cell 30,153-161.

25. Lie, W.R., Rothschild, M., and Warner, C.M. 1985. Quantitative differences in GLO enzyme levels associated with the MHC of miniature swine. Anim. Blood Grps and Biochm. Genet. 16,243-248.

26. Metzger, J.J., Lunney, J.K., Sachs, D.H., and Rudikoff, S. 1982. Transplantation in miniature swine XII. N-terminal sequences of class I histocompatibility antigens (SLA) and beta 2 microglobulin. J. Immunol. 129,716-721.

27. Osborne, B.A., Lunney, J.K., Pennington, L., Sachs, D.H., and Rudikoff, S. 1983. Two-dimensional gel analysis of swine histocompatibility antigens. J. of Immunol. 31,2939-2944.

28. Porter, R.R. 1985. The complement components coded in the

major histocompatibility complexes and their biological activities. Immunological Reviews 87, 7-17.

29. Rabin, M., Fries, R., Singer, D., and Ruddle F.H. 1985. Assignment of the porcine major histocompatibility complex to chromosome 7 by in situ hybridization. Cytogenet. Cell. Genet. 39,206-209.

30. Singer, D.S., Camerini-Otero, R.S., Satz, M.L., Osborne, B., Sachs, D., and Rudikoff, S. 1982. Characterization of a porcine genomic clone encoding a major histocompatibility antigen : expression in mouse L cells. Proc. Natl. Acad. Sci. (USA)79,1403-1407.

31. Sood, A.K., Pereira, D. and Weissman, S. 1981. Isolation and partial nucleotide sequence of a cDNA clone for human histocompatibility antigen HLA-B by use of an oligodeoxy-nucleotide primer. Proceedings of the National Academy of Science (USA) 78,616-620.

32. Southern, E.M. 1975. Detection of specific sequences among DNA fragments separated by gel electrophoresis. Journal of Molecular Biology 98,503-517.

33. Tosi, M., Levi-strauss, M., Georgatsou, E., Amor, M. and Meo,T. 1985. Duplications of complement and non-complement genes of the H-2S region : Evolutionary aspects of the C4 isotypes and molecular analysis of their expression va-riants. Immunological Reviews 87,151-184.

34. Vaiman, M., Arnoux, A., Filleul, X. and Nizza P. 1970. Le système d'histocompatibilité SLA du porc : étude par la technique des cultures mixtes de leucocytes. C.R. Acad. Sc. Paris 271,1724-1728.

35. Vaiman, M., Renard, Ch., Lafage, P., Ameteau, J. and Nizza, P. 1970. Evidence for a histocompatibility system in swine (SLA). Transplantation, 10,155-161.

36. Vaiman, M., Chardon, P., and Renard, Ch. 1979. Genetic organization of the pig SLA complex. Studies on nine recombinants and biochemical and lysostrip analysis. Immu-nogenetics 9,353-361.

37. White, P.C., New, M.I., and Dupont, B. 1985. Adrenal 21 hydroxylase cytochrome P450 genes within the MHC class III region. Immunological Reviews 87,123-150.

38. Womack, J.E., Adkison, L.R., McAvin, J.C. and Skow, L.C. 1987. Comparative gene mapping : assignment of PRGS, PAIS, IFNA, IFNB, IFNG, FN1, CRYA1, CRYG, 21OH, and the MHC to

bovine syntenic groups. 9th human gene mapping, Paris, France.

39. Yuan, P.M., Nakajin, S., Haniu, M., Shinoka, M., Hall, P.F., and Shively, J.E. 1983. Steroid 21-Hydroxylase (Cytochrome P-450) from Porcine adrenocortical microsomes: Microsequence analysis of cysteine-containing peptides. Biochemistry, 22,143-149.

40. Yuhkl, N., O'Brian, S.J. 1987. Chromosomal assignment of MHC class I and class II genes in the domestic cat, Felis 9 th human gene mapping, Paris, France.

Characterisation and Function of the Bovine MHC

R. L. Spooner, P. Brown, E. J. Glass, E. A. Innes, and J. L. Williams

Bovine MHC class I antigens can be identified
serologically with at least 30 alleles recognised
internationally as products of a single locus. MHC class
II products are less well defined by serology, whereas
alloreactive T cells and isoelectric focussing make it
possible to detect at least 12 class II alleles. The
organisation of MHC class I genes is similar to that
of man and class I cDNA shows high sequence homology
with classical MHC class I genes of man, mouse and
rabbit. Class II gene organisation also shows homology
with HLA.
Associations between BoLA and disease have been
described. It is now clear that the bovine MHC
functions in alloreactive and MHC restricted T cell
cytotoxicity and antigen presentation. Moreover immune
responses segregate in families with Class II type.
The protozoal diseases, tropical theileriosis and East
Coast fever, together with the viral disease BLV,
provide in cattle ideal models for studying a range of
immunopathological processes in an outbred species. It
is now possible to study the humoral and cellular
immune responses to potential vaccinal peptides in
cattle and attempt to overcome immune response gene
effects directly in the target animal.

The MHC in man and mouse comprises a series of closely
linked genetic loci, which are the most polymorphic
loci known. MHC gene products have been shown to play
a vital role in directing and controlling the immune
response, and can influence resistance and
susceptibility to disease (19). A knowledge of the
MHC will be necessary for the better understanding of
pathogenesis, disease susceptibility and the
development of vaccines, particularly those comprising
simple peptide antigens.

The characterisation of the MHC of domestic ruminants
may constitute a first step towards increasing the
efficiency of food production through improved disease
resistance. Once identified, useful genes can be
propagated rapidly in a population through the
application of artificial insemination, embryo
manipulation and DNA transgenic techniques.
Improvements gained through such genetic approaches
will reduce the need for sophisticated farm
management, which is of importance in third world

AFRC Inst. of Anim. Physiol. and Genet. Res., Edinburgh Res. Sta., West Mains Rd., Edinburgh EH9
3JQ, Scotland, U.K.

countries, where low input, low cost, robust systems
often have a better chance of succeeding when
intensive management and disease control systems are
prone to collapse. Even where intensive livestock
systems already exist, the potential for increased
production through reductions in sub-clinical disease
is too great to ignore.

Characterisation MHC Class I

Serology The most widely used method for studying MHC
class I polymorphism is serology. In man parous sera
are used, while in cattle alloantisera produced by
skin grafting are favoured (58).

The inheritance of serologically-defined bovine
lymphocyte antigens (BoLA) has been described (51,2)
and these have been shown to be controlled by alleles
at a single locus, the BoLA-A locus (41). A series of
international comparison tests have defined at least
30 BoLA-A locus alleles, which compares with at least
50 alleles identified serologically in the mouse (30),
however, the high frequency of null alleles (undefined)
in many cattle breeds shows that a considerable number
of bovine MHC class I gene products have yet to be
identified. As more typing reagents become available
the antigens presently characterised will, in a number
of cases, be 'split' resulting in the detection of
epitopes which are characteristic of individual gene
products. Such a splitting of A locus antigens has
been seen with the w6 specificity (55,5) and the
demonstration that w4, w7 and w10 form part of a
cross-reactive group (58). Marked differences in BoLA
gene frequencies are seen between European breeds
(43), and also between breeds throughout the world
including the tropics (28,52).

There is little serological evidence for more than one
MHC class I locus in cattle. This could be for two
reasons: tight linkage of the class I loci may result
in sera identifying haplotypes, rather than individual
products. There is some evidence for this in so far as
three workshop defined specificities are seen
together. In some breeds, e.g. in Hereford cattle,
w9, w13, w20 are often found together (R.A. Oliver
unpublished). Moreover, w25 defined in the 3rd BoLA
workshop appears to show triplets with several
specificities. Also not all European sera work as well
in West Africa (52) or East Africa (28) as in Europe,
for example, only 6.4 behaves as a true w6 subgroup.
These examples may reflect recombination between MHC

class I loci which have been fixed in the different
breeds. The sera produced in cattle may also identify
only the most antigenic locus.

Monoclonal Antibody Definition of Class I gene
products Although alloantisera have been the basic
tools for bovine class I antigen definition,
monoclonal antibodies have the advantage that they see
individual epitopes and that they can be produced in
large quantities. Several monoclonal antibodies (mAbs)
detecting epitopes on class I antigens of other
species have been tested with bovine cells, but most
detect non-polymorphic determinants (11). Hitherto
only a limited number of mAbs which define bovine
class I polymorphism have been reported
(56,64,16,65,66). It is nevertheless likely, that
interest in the development of such reagents will be
maintained. Evidence for other expressed MHC class I
loci in cattle has been obtained from the sequential
precipitation with several polymorphic bovine MHC
class I monoclonal antibodies and the non-polymorphic
human MHC class I monoclonal antibody, W6/32. Such an
approach suggests that in excess of 4 different MHC
class I antigens are found on the bovine cell surface
(A. Bensaid and A.J Teale unpublished), although
these preliminary results are open to the criticism
that each precipitation may be incomplete.

T cell cytotoxicity   In the characterisation of
the human MHC antigens, alloreactive cytotoxic T
lymphocytes (CTL) have been useful in detecting
subtypes of serologically-defined class I antigen
specificities (25,49). In cattle serologically defined
subtypes also function as target antigens for
alloreactive T cells, whereas the supertypic
specificities do not(64,59). There is thus better
correlation between the CTL and serological
definitions of BoLA specificities than is found in
man.

The derivation of alloreactive T lymphocyte clones
specific for bovine class I antigens has recently been
described (65). While not useful as tools for routine
typing, cloned T cells can be of use in fine
dissection of selected haplotypes.

MHC Class I Genes   A molecular biological approach
to the bovine MHC has also been used in the attempt to
define the number of class I loci in cattle. A bovine
class I cDNA (cBOLA-1) has been isolated from a liver
cDNA library (P Brown unpublished). This cDNA has been

completely sequenced and codes for a protein of 339
amino acid residues. It compared well with other
classical MHC class I proteins which vary in length
from 339 amino acids for HLA-B7 to 348 residues for H-
2K^b (29). The deduced amino acid sequence has been
compared with MHC class I sequences from rat, mouse,
rabbit and man and retains protein modification sites
at the correct locations and cysteine residues
correctly positioned for the formation of internal
disulphide bridges. We thus infer that cBoLA-1
represents functional BoLA class I mRNA. Regions of
variation between published MHC class I protein
sequences and cBOLA-1 occur clustered in the protein
domain that is proposed to form the antigen binding
site (9,10).

The bovine cDNA has been used to probe bovine genomic
Southern blots and reveals in excess of 12 fragments
per animal with different restriction enzymes,
indicating that multiple MHC class I sequences are present
in the bovine genome as with man, rat, horse and mice
(14,61,8). Several fragments are highly polymorphic
and in some cases can be correlated with serological
specificities in unrelated animals. The bovine MHC
class I region therefore is multigenic, and the
polymorphic fragments may code for classical MHC class
I genes while the non-polymorphic fragments code genes
similar to the conserved Qa or TLA genes of the mouse.
Restriction fragment length polymorphism has been used
to identify MHC class I types in man (17) but is by no
means as far advanced in cattle.

Mutants deleted for particular MHC class I antigens
have been described (A.J. Teale unpublished). DNA
from these mutants has been probed with cBOLA-1 in
attempt to correlate fragments with loss of expression
(P.Brown and A.Teale unpublished). A similar approach
has been described for man (43) the results from
cattle are encouraging with definite loss of
hybridising bands.

Characterisation of MHC Class II

Serology   Relatively little is known of MHC class
II antigens of cattle; this is largely due to the lack
of a suitable serological test. There are three
principal reasons for this. First, class II antigens
are only expressed on around 30% of a normal PBM
population, second, most alloantisera possess anti-
class I reactivity which must be removed before class
II definition can be undertaken. This can be achieved

by absorption with platelets and although the
technique is tedious some useful sera have been
reported (20,M.J. Stear unpublished). A third reason
may be that class II antigens are less antigenic than
class I.

A number of mAbs raised against MHC class II antigens
of other species react with bovine class II products
(57,35) and mAbs have been raised against the bovine
antigens themselves (33,31). However, none has so far
been shown to detect polymorphism.

T lymphocyte reactivity   In view of the
difficulties involved in serotyping bovine class II
antigens, the use of cellular techniques has received
greater emphasis. Using mixed lymphocyte reactions
(MLR), in which T cells mount a proliferative response
to non-self class II antigens, evidence was obtained
suggesting significant polymorphism in bovine class II
antigens (68,18). Further MLR studies,using full sib
families, demonstrated that the genes controlling the
MLR were linked to the class I antigens (51,68).

As with serotyping methods for class II antigens, the
MLR has not been widely used, due in part to the poor
repeatability of results. Recently the development of
alloreactive bovine T cell clones has been reported
(65) and their use in the detection of class II
antigen polymorphisms described (66). Such T cell
clones, characterised by the BoT4+ phenotype, mount
reliable responses.in proliferation assays. Their use
is therefore not subject to the constraints affecting
the standard MLR. They will probably be particularly
appropriate for the definition of functionally
important epitopes on MHC class II molecules, as in
other species (47).

MHC Class II Genes   The genes coding for the bovine
MHC class II antigens have been studied by the cross
hybridisation of human MHC class II cDNA probes on
genomic Southern blots. There is strong evidence for
HLA DQ and DR like loci in cattle, with several α and
β genes at each locus (3).The DQ and DR like loci are
highly polymorphic and in strong linkage
disequilibrium (4). There is also evidence for a DP
like locus in cattle (J. L. Williams and A. Bensaid
unpublished), however other workers fail to see
hybridisation of HLA DP probes to bovine DNA. Field
inversion gel electrophoresis has shown that the
bovine MHC class II region is contained within 1.5
mega bases of DNA (Bensaid unpublished). There is no

information on the number of functional genes at each
locus and complete genomic definition of the bovine
MHC region awaits the characterisation of overlapping
genomic clones.

Isoelectric focussing

The use of isoelectric focussing of MHC Class I and
Class II products after immunoprecipitation and
neuraminidase treatment has been used to identify MHC
antigens in man (40). This method has now been applied
to cattle for identifying both BoLA Class I and Class
II phenotypes (E. Hensen and R.L. Spooner unpublished).
For MHC class I antigens the correlation with serology
is very good and the method makes it possible to
identify MHC antigens where appropriate alloantisera
are not available. For MHC Class I two or three bands
are seen on the IEF gels for each haplotype, which may
indicate that there is more than one expressed Class I
locus in cattle. This is further suggested by IEF
analysis of the products precipitated by different
monoclonal antibodies. However, until peptide mapping
has been completed this cannot be confirmed.

This is the first method to be described whereby the
products of MHC class II haplotypes can be identified
in cattle. In a study using a limited number of
animals, 12 different MHC class II haplotypes have
been identified, demonstrating the high degree of
polymorphism in the population(E. Hensen, R.A. Oliver
and J.L. Williams unpublished). Comparison of the MHC
class II types identified by IEF in unrelated animals
of given class I type shows that there is high linkage
disequilibrium between the two loci.

An alternative approach is the isoelectric focusing of
unprecipitated,solubilised membrane proteins which can
then be transferred onto nitrocellulose filters. The
MHC class I or class II products can then be detected
with suitable monoclonal antibodies or antisera to
monomorphic determinants. Such a western blotting
system has been used to identify polymorphism of MHC
Class II products in cattle (J.L. Williams
unpublished).

Immune responsiveness

In mice the association of antigen with surface
MHC molecules has been shown to be essential for
recognition of antigen and subsequent generation of an
antigen specific immune response. Congenic mice with

the IA^d MHC type are able to respond to ovalbumin peptides, while mice with IA^k are not. This has been shown to be due to differing affinities of these MHC molecules for ovalbumin (7).

Several studies have indicated that the bovine MHC class I and class II antigens have similar function. Cattle immunised with HSA and (T,G)-A--L show significant differences in immune response for different BoLA types, BoLA-w16 was associated with high response to HSA and BoLA-w2 with low response (36).BoLA w16 has been shown to be in very strong linkage disequilibrium with MHC class II (L. Anderson unpublished).It is of interest to note that an earlier study demonstrated that high HSA response was associated with susceptibility to mastitis.

An in vitro T cell proliferation assay has been developed to investigate immune response to antigen in cattle (23) and has demonstrated that T cell proliferation is dependent on antigen presenting cells and can be inhibited by anti-MHC class II antibodies. Following immunisation with ovalbumin cattle can be divided into those showing a T cell proliferative response and those that do not . Interestingly there is an inverse relationship between T cell proliferation and humoral response. The type of response segregates with Class II haplotype in families (E. J. Glass, J. L. Williams and E. Hensen unpublished).

Cytotoxic cells and Class I Serologically defined bovine MHC Class I products have been shown to be the principal recognition structures for alloreactive bovine T cell lines and clones (63,64,59). They also act as restriction elements in cytotoxic responses against pathogen infected host cells. This classical MHC restriction of bovine cytotoxic cells has been elegantly demonstrated using the Theileria model. Theileria parva and Theileria annulata are two closely related protozoan parasites that infect the lymphocytes of cattle and African buffalos. As in the case with certain viral infections, the parasite causes antigenic changes on the cell surface, against which the host mounts a cytotoxic T cell response. An early indication that this CTL response may be genetically restricted was in a study described by Eugie and Emery (22) in which they demonstrated that CTL from immune cattle would preferentially kill autologous Theileria infected target cells in-vitro. Further studies using BoLA defined cattle have shown

that MHC restricted cytotoxic cells are generated in
vivo in cattle immune to either T. parva (39, 24) or T.
annulata (27, 46). Theileria-specific CTL clones have
recently been generated and characterised both
phenotypically and functionally. These cytotoxic
effectors were of the BoT8 phenotype (bovine
equivalent of CD8) and exhibited genetic restriction
which correlated with the recognition of MHC Class I A
locus specificities. The cytotoxic response was
inhibited by the addition of the appropriate Class I
alloantisera by the mAb w6/32 (24) which reacts with a
non-polymorphic determinant on bovine Class I
molecules (16). Interestingly, it was observed that
the CTL response, in cattle that were heterozygous at
the BoLA Class I A locus, was strongly biased towards
one of the alleles (38).

Theileria infected cell line immunisation   Role of
the MHC. A unique feature of Theileria parasites is
their ability to infect bovine mononuclear cells
resulting in the synchronous division of parasite and
host cells. The property of these infected cells
allows them to be maintained indefinitely in vitro as
persistently infected lymphoblastoid cell lines,
without the addition of exogenous growth factors (13)
These cell lines when inoculated into susceptible
cattle can induce protection although the system is
complicated by the problem of histoincompatibility;
whereby the cell line vaccine effectively introduces
the parasite to the recipient animal in the context of
a foreign graft. However T. annulata infected cell
lines behave differently than T. parva cell lines since
very high doses of allogeneic T. parva infected cell
lines,(10^8 cells or more) are required to reproducibly
infect animals (13). When lower cell doses are used T.
parva is only transmissable if the cell line is
autologous or BoLA matched to the recipient (62,21).
In contrast it is possible to infect and immunise
animals with as few as 10^2 allogeneic T. annulata
infected cells (26). It was assumed that the problem
in the case of T. parva was one of
histoincompatibility whereby the allogeneic cell line
was simply rejected before parasite infection of the
host cells could take place. However, a cellular
graft rejection response specific for the bovine MHC
Class I products present on the donor cell line has
recently been demonstrated in allogeneic T. annulata
cell line immunisation, and these animals were fully
protected against challenge (27). Therefore this
difference in ease of allogeneic cell line
immunisation between T. parva and T. annulata cannot

simply be explained by a graft rejection phenomenon.

Disease Associations

In man where MHC class I and class II antigens can be
defined reliably, there is still only a limited
amount of information about the involvement of the MHC
in disease resistance. For autoimmune diseases strong
associations have been described with particular MHC
class II antigens, e.g. DR4 is associated with insulin
dependent diabetes. There is even less data on the
role of the MHC in regulating immune response to
infectious dieases. DR4 or DR6 have been implicated in
susceptibility to cholera and yellow fever.

Bovine leukaemia virus infection in a herd of
Shorthorn cattle, where 51% of the animals were
seropositive and 23% of the seropositive cows were
lymphocytotoxic, suggested an association between BoLA
and susceptibility/resistance to subclinical, B-cell
proliferative stages of BLV infection (36). The
offspring of a bull, heterozygous for susceptibility
and resistance, which received the susceptibility
allele and also BoLA w8.1 from their dams, showed
greater B cell proliferation and lymphocytosis, than
those that had not received w8.1. However in another
family in Holsteins w8.1 was associated with lower B
cell numbers (H.A. Lewin, unpublished) These results
would indicate that the subclinical progression of BLV
is in part controlled by genes in the bovine MHC.
Furthermore, since the same class I allele (w8.1) was
associated with susceptibility in one breed and
resistance in another, a role for class II genes is
suggested since it is likely that different haplotypes
exist in the two breeds.

BoLA-w16 has been implicated in susceptibility to
mastitis and BoLA-w2 with resistance in Norwegian
cattle (50). BoLA-w16 is tightly linked to the red
cell antigen M (34),and significantly, evidence of
association between blood group M and susceptibility
to mastitis has been reported (32). Correlation of
BoLA alleles with mastitis susceptibility and mastitis
related traits, such as milk cell counts, ATP and
antitrypsin levels, has also been made in Icelandic
cattle (42). BoLA-w6 and w6.1 were associated with
high cell counts and w6.2, w11, ED085 and ED109 with
high antitrypsin levels. The class I determinant
detected by mAb ILA-A7, showed a significant
association with low cell counts. Unfortunately w16
and w2, the extreme alleles found in the Norwegian

study (50), were not present in the Icelandic
population.

There are considerable differences between breeds and
individuals within breeds in the level of infestation
with ticks and this is a heritable trait (69). In
Australia BoLA-w6 has been associated with the highest
levels of infestation (60). However, it is not known
whether this is due to the MHC antigens or to other
genes encoded within the MHC, e.g. 21-hydroxylase.

The BoLA w6 has also been associated with
susceptibility to cancer eye in Herefords (M.J. Stear
unpublished); nevertheless w6 is found in high
frequency in many populations and care must taken to
avoid making associations with the most frequent
alleles.Evidence has been presented that w6 is
associated with an increased twinning rate (M.J. Stear
unpublished) which could explain why an apparently
disadvantagous allele is maintained at a high
frequency.

Conclusions.

Cattle are an important source of food worldwide thus
understanding their physiological and pathological
processes is essential for improving productivity. In
addition cattle are subject to diseases which are good
models for disease in man and other species. For
example, bovine theileriosis is a good model for the
study of T cell mediated immune response and leucocyte
transformation by protozoan infection and BLV an
excellent model for HTLV-1 infection.

Although early studies of the ruminant MHC systems
were dependent on serological definition of MHC class
I antigens, the recent development of T cell assays
and of biochemical and DNA technology has enabled
better definition of MHC class I and class II types.
The anticipated cloning of ruminant MHC genes should
considerably assist definition of the MHC at the genome
level and may provide tools for the production of
monoclonal antibodies recognising polymorphism in
bovine MHC antigens. In addition allele-specific
oligonucleotides can then be made which will allow
rapid and precise DNA typing of MHC phenotypes. It
should be stressed, however, that definition of MHC
products by the established serological, cellular and
biochemical approaches are a means of defining
expressed, functionally relevant antigens.

The role of the MHC in mediating different facets of
the immune response has been most clearly demonstrated
in the murine and human systems; studies in cattle
strongly support the ruminant MHC having an equally
important function. With the increasing definition of
the MHC of domestic ruminants we can envisage the
identification of individual genes which improve the
level of the immune response either in general, or to
specific pathogens. The dissemination of such genes to
certain populations by large scale artificial
insemination, embryo manipulation or DNA transgenic
techniques, could bestow increased fitness of those
populations in particular environments.

Such genetic improvement would be invaluable
economically, particularly if strong MHC associations
are found with major diseases in developed or
developing countries.

Considerable effort has already been made towards the
characterisation of the ruminant MHC, and the
application of modern technology should allow rapid
progress.

REFERENCES

1.   Alexander, A.J., Bailey, E. & Woodward, J.G.
(1987).   Analysis of Equine Lymphocyte Antigen system
by Southern blot hybridisation.   Immunogenetics, 25,
47-54.

2.   Amorena, B. & Stone, W.H. (1978). Serologically
defined (SD) locus in cattle. Science, 201, 159-160.

3.   Andersson, L., Bohme, J., Rask, L. & Peterson,
P.A.   (1986b).   Genomic hybridisation of bovine
Class II major histocompatibility genes.   I.
Extensive polymorphism of DQa and DQB genes.   Anim.
Genet. 17: 95-112.

4.   Andersson, L., Bohme, J., Peterson, P.A. & Rask,
L.   (1986a).   Genomic hybridization of bovine Class
II major histocompatability genes.   II. Polymorphism
of DR genes and linkage disequilibrium in the DQ-DR
region.   Anim. Genet. 17: 295-304.

5.   Anon. Proceedings of the Second International
Bovine Lymphocyte (BoLA) Workshop. (1982). Animal
Blood Groups and Biochemical Genetics, 3, 33-53.

6.   Anon. Proceedings of the Third International BoLA workshop. (1987). Animal Genetics, (in preparation).

7.   Babbitt, D.P., Allen, P.M., Matsueda, G., Haber, E. and Unanue, E.R., (1985). Binding of immunogenic peptides to Ia histocompatibility molecules. Nature 317, 359-361.

8.   Biro, P.A., Par, J., Sood, A.K., Kole, R., Reddy, V.B. & Weissmal, S.M.   (1983).   The Major Histocompatibility complex. Cold Spring Harbour Symposium, Quantitative Biology, 47: 1079-1086.

9.   Bjorkman, P.J., Saper, M.A., Samraoui, B., Bennett, W.S., Strominger, J.L. & Wiley, D.C. (1987). Structure of the human Class I histocompatibility antigen. HLA-A2.   Nature, 329, 506-512.

10.   Bjorkman, P.J., Saper, M.A., Samraoui, B., Bennett, W.S., Strominger, J.L. & Wiley, D.C. (1987).   The foreign antigen binding site and T cell recognition regions of Class I histocompatibility antigens.   Nature, 329: 512-518.

11.   Brodsky, F.M., Stone, W.H. & Parham, P. (1981). Of cows and men: A comparative study of histocompatibility antigens. Human Immunology, 3, 143-152.

12.   Brown, C.G.D., Malmquist, W.A., Cunningham, M.P. & Burridge, M.J. (1971). Immunisation against East Coast fever. Inoculation of cattle with Theileria parva schizonts grown in cell culture. Journal of Parasitology, 57, 59-60.

13.   Brown, C.G.D., Crawford, J.G., Kanhai, G.K., Njuguna, L.M. & Stagg, D.A. (1978). Immunization of cattle against East Coast fever with lymphoblastoid cell lines infected and transformed by Theileria parva, in "Tick-borne Diseases and their Vectors", (ed. J.K.H. Wilde), University of Edinburgh, 331-335.

14.   Cami, B., Bregegere, F., Abastado, P. & Kowrilsky, P. (1981). Multiple sequences related to classical histocompatibility antigens in the mouse genome.   Nature 291: 673-675.

15.   Chardon, M., Vaiman, M., Kirzenbaum, M.,
Geffrotin, C. Renard, C. & Cohen, D. (1985). Studies
of MHC in farm animals by restriction enzyme
polymorphism. Animal Blood Groups and Biochemical
Genetics, 16, Suppl 1, 121-122.

16.   Chardon, P., Kali, J., Leveziel, H., Colombani,
J. & Vaiman, M. (1983). Monoclonal antibodies to HLA
recognize monomorphic and polymorphic epitopes on
BoLA. Tissue Antigens, 22, 62-71.

17.   Cohen, D., Paul, P., Le Gall, I., Marcadet, A.,
Font, M.P., Cohen-Hageunauer, O., Sayagh, B., Cann,
H., Lalovel, J.M. and Dausset, J.   (1985).   DNA
Polymorphism of HLA Class I and Class II regions.
Immunological Reviews 85: 87-105.

18.   Curie-Cohen, M., Usinger, W.R. & Stone, W.H.
(1978). Transitivity of response in the mixed
lymphocyte culture test. Tissue Antigens, 12, 170-178.

19.   Dausset, J. & Svejgaard, A. (1978). HLA and
Disease, (eds.J. Dausset and A. Svejgaard),
Munksgaard, Copenhagen.

20.   Davies, C.J. and Antczak, D.F. (1987). Serological
and cellular typing for bovine class II antigens
reveals complexity in the bovine MHC.   Animal Genetics,
18, Suppl 1, 13-14.

21.   Dolan, T.T., Teale, A.J., Stagg, D.A., Kemp,
S.J., Cowan, K.M., Young, A.S., Groocock, C.M.,
Leitch, B.L., Spooner, R.L. & Brown, C.D.G. (1984). A
histocompatibility barrier to immunization against
East Coast fever using Theileria parva-infected
lymphoblastoid cell lines. Parasite Immunology, 6,
243-250.

22.   Eugie, E.M. & Emery, D.L. (1981). Genetically
restricted cell-mediated cytotoxicity in cattle immune
to Theileria parva. Nature, 290, 251-254.

23.   Glass, E.J. and Spooner, R.L. (1988). Requirement
for MHC class II positive accessory cells in an
antigen specific bovine T cell response. Immunology
(submitted).

24.   Goddeeris, B.M., Morrison, W.I., Teale, A.J.,
Bensaid, A. & Baldwin, C.L. (1986). Bovine cytotoxic T
cell clones specific for cells infected with the
protozoan parasite Theileria parva: Parasite strain
specificity and class I MHC restriction. Proceedings
of the National Academy of Sciences (U.S.A), 83, 5238-
5242.

25.   Horai, S., Poel, J.J. van der. & Goulmy, E.
(1982). Differential recognition of the serologically
defined HLA-A2 antigen by allogeneic cytotoxic T-
cells. I. Population studies. Immunogenetics, 16, 135-
142.

26.   Innes, E.A., Ouhelli, H., Oliver, R.A., Brown,
C.G.D. & Spooner, R.L.   The effect of MHC
compatibility between parasite infected cell line and
recipient in immunisation against tropical
Theileriosis.   Parasite Immunology.   (Submitted).

27.   Innes, E.A., Miller, P., Preston, P.M., Brown,
C.G.D. & Spooner, R.L.   The specificity of cytotoxic
cells in cattle immunised with autologous and
allogenic lymphoblastoid cell lines infected and
transformed by a Moroccan strain of T. annulata.
European Journal of Immunology. (Submitted).

28.   Kemp, S.J., Spooner, R.L. & Teale, A.J.   (1988).
MHC of African and European cattle. Animal Genetics 19
In Press.

29.   Kimball, E.S. & Coligan, J.E.   (1983).
Structure of Class I Major Histocompatibility
Antigens.   Contemporary Topics Molecular Immunology,
9: 1-63.

30.   Klein, J.   (1979).   The Major Histocompatibility
complex of the Mouse.   Science, 203: 516-521.

31.   Lalor, P.A., Morrison, W.I., Goddeeris, B.M.,
Jack, R.M. & Black, S.J. (1986). Monoclonal antibodies
identify phenotypically and functionally distinct cell
types in the bovine lymphoid system. Veterinary
Immunology and Immunopathology, 13, 121-140.

32.   Larsen, B., Jensen, N.E., Madsen, P., Nielsen,
S.M., Klastrup, O. & Madsen, P.S. (1985).Association
of the M blood group system with bovine mastitis.
Animal Blood Groups & Biochemical Genetics, 16, 165-
173.

33.   Letesson, J.J., Coppe, Ph., Lostrie-Trussart, N.
& Depelchin, A. (1983). A bovine Ia-like antigen
detected by a xenogeneic monoclonal antibody. Animal
Blood Groups and Biochemical Genetics, 14, 239-250.

34.   Leveziel, H. & Hines, H.C. (1984). Linkage in
cattle between the major histocompatibility complex
(BoLA) and the M blood group system. Genetique
Selection et Evolution, 16, 405-416,

35.   Lewin, H.A., Davis, W.C. & Bernoco, D. (1985).
Monoclonal antibodies that recognize bovine T and B
lymphocytes. Veterinary Immunology and
Immunopathology, 9, 87-102.

36.   Lewin, H.A. & Bernoco, D. (1986). Evidence for
BoLA-linked resistance and susceptibility to
subclinical progression of bovine leukaemia virus
infection. Animal Genetics, 17, 197-208.

37.   Lie, O., Solbu, H., Larsen, H.J. & Spooner, R.L.
(1986). Evidence for MHC control of immune
responsiveness in cattle. Veterinary Immunology &
Immunopathology, 11, 333-350.

38.   Morrison, W.I., Emery, D.L., Teale, A.J. &
Goddeeris, B.M. (1986a). Protective immune responses
in bovine theileriosis.In 'The Ruminant Immune System
in Health and Disease', (ed. W.I.Morrison), Cambridge
University Press, 555-570.

39.   Morrison, W.I., Goddeeris, B.M., Teale, A.J.,
Baldwin, C.L., Bensaid, A. & Ellis, J. (1986b). Cell-
mediated immune responses of cattle and their role in
immunity to the protozoan parasite Theileria parva.
Immunology Today, 7, 211-213.

40.   Neefjes, J.J., Doxiadis, I., Stam, N.J. Beckers,
C.J. & Ploegh, H.L. (1986). An analysis of Class I
Antigens of Man and other species by one-dimensional
IEF and Immunoblotting. Immunogenetics 23: 164-171.

41.   Newman, M.J., Adams, T.E; & Brandon, M.R. (1982).
Serological and genetic identification of a bovine B
lymphocyte alloantigen system. Animal Blood Groups and
Biochemical Genetics, 13, 123-129.

42.   Oddgeirsson,O., Simpson,S.P.,Ross,D.S. & Spooner,
R.L. (1988) Relationship between the bovine MHC (BoLA)
and mastitis, cell count, ATP and antitrypsin levels
in Icelandic cattle. Animal Genetics, 18 (In Press).

43   Oliver, R.A., McCoubrey, C.M., Millar, P.,
Morgan, A.L.G. & Spooner, R.L. (1981). A genetic study
of bovine lymphocyte antigens (BoLA) and their
frequency in several breeds. Immunogenetics, 13, 127-
132.

44.   Orr, H.T., Bach, F.H., Ploegh, H.L., Strominger,
J.L., Kavathas, P. and Demars, R.   (1982).   Use of
HLA loss mutants to analyse the structure of the human
major histocompatibility complex. Nature 296, 454-
456.

45.   Palmer, M., Wettstein, P.J. & Frelinger, J.A.
(1983). Evidence for extensive polymorphism of Class I
genes in the rat major histocompatibility complex
(RT1).   Immunology, 80: 7616-7620.

46.   Preston, P.M., Brown, C.G.D. & Spooner, R.L.
(1983). Cell-mediated cytotoxicity in Theileria
annulata infection of cattle with evidence for BoLA
restriction. Clinical and Experimental Immunology, 53,
88-100.

47.   Rosen-Bronson, S., Johnson, A.H., Hartzman, R.J.
& Eckels, D.D. (1986). Human allospecific TLCs
generated against HLA antigens associated with DR1
through DRw8. Immunogenetics, 23, 368-378.

48.   Schwartz, R.D.   (1980).   Immune response (Ir)
genes of the murine major histocompatibility complex.
Adv. Immunol., 38: 31.

49.   Spits, H., Breuning, M.H., Ivanyi, P., Russo, C.
& Vries, J.E. de. (1982). In vitro-isolated human
cytotoxic T-lymphocyte clones detect variation in
serologically defined HLA antigens. Immunogenetics,
16, 503-512.

50.   Solbu, H., Spooner, R.L. & Lie, O. (1982). A
possible influence of the bovine major
histocompatibility Complex (BoLA) on mastitis.
Proceedings of 2nd World Congress on Genetics applied
to Livestock Production, Madrid. 1-6.

51.   Spooner, R.L., Leveziel, H., Grosclaude. F.,
Oliver, R.A. & Vaiman, M. (1978). Evidence for a
possible major histocompatibility complex (BoLA) in
cattle. Journal of Immunogenetics, 5, 335-346.

52.   Spooner, R.L., Leveziel, H., Queval, R. & Hoste,
C. (1987). Studies on the histocompatibility complex
of indigenous cattle in the Ivory Coast. Veterinary
Immunology and Immunopathology, 15, 377-384.

53.   Spooner, R.L., Oliver, R.A., Sales, D.I.,
McCoubrey, C.M., Millar, P., Morgan, A.G., Amorena,
B., Bailey, E., Bernoco, D., Brandon, M., Bull, R.W.,
Caldwell, J., Cwik, S., van Dam, R.H., Dodd, J.,
Gahne, B., Grosclaude, F., Hall, J.G., Hines, H.,
Leveziel, H., Newman, M., Stear, M.J., Stone, W.H. &
Vaiman, M. (1979). Analysis of alloantisera against
bovine lymphocytes. Joint Report of the 2nd
International Bovine Lymphocyte Antigen (BoLA)
Workshop. Animal Blood Groups and Biochemical
Genetics, 10, 63-68.

54.   Spooner, R.L. & Brown, C.G.D. (1980). Bovine
lymphocyte antigens (BoLA) of bovine lymphocytes and
derived lymphoblastoid lines transformed by Theileria
parva and Theileria annulata. Parasite Immunology, 2,
163-174.

55.   Spooner, R.L. & Morgan, A.L.G. (1981). Analysis
of BoLA w6. Evidence for multiple subgroups. Tissue
Antigens, 17, 178-188.

56.   Spooner, R.L. & Pinder, M. (1983). Monoclonal
antibodies to bovine MHC products. Veterinary
Immunology and Immunopathology, 4, 453-458. .

57.   Spooner, R.L. & Ferrone, S. (1984). Cross
reaction of monoclonal antibodies to human MHC Class I
and Class II products with bovine lymphocyte
subpopulations. Tissue Antigens, 24, 270-277.

58.   Spooner, R.L. (1986). The bovine major
histocompatibility complex. In 'The Ruminant Immune
System in Health and Disease', (ed. W.I. Morrison),
Cambridge University Press, Cambridge, 133-151.

59.   Spooner, R.L., Innes, E.A., Millar, P., Webster,
J. & Teale, A.J. (1987). Bovine alloreactive cytotoxic
cells generated in vitro detect BoLA w6 subgroups.
Immunology, 61, 85-91.

60.   Stear, M.J., Newman, M.J., Nicholas, F.W., Brown,
S.C. & Holroyd, R.G. (1984). Tick resistance and the
bovine major histocompatibility system. Australian
Journal of Experimental Biology and Medical
Science, 62, 47-52.

61.   Steinmetz, M., Frelinger, J.G., Fisher, D., Hunkapiller, T., Pereira, D., Weissman, S.M., Uehara, H., Nathenson, S. & Hood, L.   (1981).   Three cDNA clones encoding mouse transplantation antigens: Homology to immunoglobulin genes.   Cell, 24: 125-134.

62.   Teale, A.J. (1983). The major histocompatibility complex of cattle with particular reference to some aspects of East Coast fever. Ph.D. Thesis, University of Edinburgh.

63.   Teale, A.J., Morrison, W.I., Goddeeris, B.M., Groocock, C.M., Stagg, D.A. & Spooner, R.L. (1985). Bovine alloreactive cytotoxic cells generated in vitro: target specificity in relation to BoLA phenotype. Immunology, 55, 355-362.

64.   Teale, A.J., Morrison, W.I., Spooner, R.L., Goddeeris, B.M., Groocock, C.M. & Stagg, D.A.   Bovine alloreactive cytotoxic T cells. (1986a). In 'The Ruminant Immune System in Health and Disease', (ed. W.I. Morrison), Cambridge University Press, 322-345.

65.   Teale, A.J., Baldwin, C.L., Ellis, J.A., Newson, J., Goddeeris, B.M. & Morrison, W.I. (1986b). Alloreactive bovine T Lymphocyte clones: An analysis of function, phenotype and specificity. Journal of Immunology, 136, 4392-4398.

66.   Teale, A.J. & Kemp, S.J. (1987). A study of BoLA class II antigens with Bo T4+ T lymphocyte clones. Animal Genetics, 18, 17-28.

67.   Usinger, W.R., Curie-Cohen, H. & Stone, W.H. (1977). Lymphocyte-defined loci in cattle. Science, 196, 1017-1018.

68.   Usinger, W.R., Curie-Cohen, M., Benforado, K., Pringnitz, D., Rowe, R., Splitter, G.A. & Stone, W.H. (1981). The bovine major histocompatibility complex (BoLA): Close linkage of the genes controlling serologically-defined antigens and mixed lymphocyte reactivity. Immunogenetics, 14, 423-428.

69.   Wagland, B.M.   (1975).   Host resistance to the cattle tick (Boophilus microplus) in Brahmin (Bos indicus) cattle.   1. Responses of previously unexposed cattle to four infestations with 20,000 larvae. Aust. agric. 26: 1073-1080.

7 SLA Monoclonal Antibodies

Joan K. Lunney, Donald C. Sun, Diana Ivanoska, Mark D. Pescovitz, and William C. Davis

Traditionally alloantisera have been the reagents of choice for detecting alleles of MHC antigens. With the advent of monoclonal antibody (mAb) technology we and others began to produce mAb to SLA antigens. SLA class I mAb were identified by their reactivity with >90% of PBMC, by binding to SLA class I gene transfected L cells and by their antigen MW. We have produced several new mAb reactive with monomorphic SLA class I determinants as well as mAb reactive with allelic determinant(s) of the PD14 SLA class I gene product. MAb to class II SLA antigens have been easier to find because of the extensive interspecies cross reactions. Mouse anti-I-E mAb were first shown by us to be reactive with a subset of SLA class II antigens and designated as the SLA-DRw antigens. More recently we have demonstrated a second lower MW subset of class II antigens using mAb against bovine class II antigens and designated them as the SLA-DQw antigens. There are however still very few mAb that recognize allelic determinants of SLA class II antigens. MAb to SLA antigens are only tools to analyze the genetic complexity of immune responses and regulation; specific examples of such uses will be covered in the final part of this chapter.

A. BACKGROUND

The importance of MHC antigens was indicated by the early work of McDevitt, Benacerraf, and others who proved that immune responses to simple foreign antigens were controlled by genes that coded for the class II antigens of the MHC complex (1, 2). The significance of these basic findings, that responder phenotype is dependent on host genetic inheritance, has been reinforced by the recent failures of trials of the malaria peptide vaccine in human volunteers (3). In control tests, the peptide vaccine stimulated positive antibody responses only in some individuals, i.e., in those who inherited particular alleles at the MHC class II loci (4). In addition this vaccine is also missing epitopes that stimulate the proliferative, immune enhancing T cell component necessary for high level vaccine responses (5). Taken together these results with the malaria peptide vaccine demonstrate how important basic immune response gene research is for designing effective

Lunney and Sun: Helminthic Dis. Lab., LPSI, Bldg. 1040, BARC-East, ARS, USDA, Beltsville, Md. Ivanoska: INEP, Zemun, Yugoslavia. Pescovitz: Dept. of Surg., Univ. of Minn. Med. Sch., Minneapolis, Minn. Davis: Dept. of Vet. Microbiol. and Path., Wash. State Univ., Pullman, Wash.

vaccines against pathogens, and reinforce the usefulness of MHC typing reagents in determining the genetic complexity of target livestock populations for vaccine trials. Many disease responses are also regulated by MHC determined interactions as evidenced most recently by the demonstration that transgenic progeny of mice who were susceptible to diabetes could be made resistant to that disease by the introduction of a specific MHC class II gene into their DNA (6).

The existence of the swine MHC or SLA (swine leukocyte antigen) complex was clearly established by Vaiman and Binns and their colleagues (7, 8). Vaiman et al. (9) and Lunney et al. (10) demonstrated the role of SLA antigens in regulating immune responses to small antigens. Serum titers following vaccination with Bordetella bronchiseptica and modified pseudorabies virus, as well as muscle larval burdens after Trichinella spiralis infections, also appear to be regulated by genes within this complex (11-14). In addition, genetic influences on ovulation rate and on certain production traits correlate with inheritance of certain haplotypes of the SLA complex (15-19).

The SLA complex is a set of linked genes that encode the class I and class II SLA glycoproteins. The traditional class I genes are designated SLA-A,B,C and encode 45,000d glycoproteins that noncovalently associate with 12,000d β_2-microglobulin on the cell surface of most cells (20, 21). It is expected that the SLA complex will also encode the Qa and Tla equivalent, class I-like differentiation antigens of swine. Based on data in other species, these antigens are expected to be about 40,000d proteins and to be expressed only on subsets of differentiated cells (22). The SLA class II genes encode the SLA-DR,DQ and, if expressed, DP antigens, consisting of 33-35,000d alpha chains associated with 27-28,000d beta chains (21, 23, 24). In swine, the class II antigens are expressed on all B cells, on macrophages, and unexpectedly on certain subsets of T cells (25-27).

As noted in other papers in this volume, the MHC antigens are unusual in that they are extraordinarily polymorphic. There may be over 50 alleles at any one locus (28); in addition, alleles at the same locus may differ by as much as 40% in their amino acid sequences (29, 30). Restriction fragment length polymorphism (RFLP) analysis of genomic DNA has demonstrated that any one individual pig chromosome encodes between 7 and 10 class I-like genes (31-34). Although this is among the smallest number of class I genes in any species, the major expressed genes are the traditional class I antigens, the SLA A,B,C antigens. Singer's laboratory has cloned 7 SLA class I genes; two of these, PD1 and PD14, can be expressed after transfection into L cells and may encode SLA-A,B,C antigens (32). A third gene, PD6, is a good candidate for a Qa2-like gene because of its preferential transcription in T cells, no cell surface antigen has yet been detected in PD6 transfected L cells (35). RFLP analysis of SLA class II DNA has revealed at least 3 alpha chain genes and 5-8 beta chain genes for each chromosome bearing the SLA complex (33, 34, 36, 37). Preliminary evidence indicates that there is no gene to encode the SLA-DP alpha protein (Sachs et al., personal communication). As will be discussed below, there is clear biochemical evidence for cell surface expression of at least SLA-DRw and SLA-DQw antigens on pig PBMC (38, 39).

Because of the complexity of the MHC, and of the importance of the SLA complex in determining a wide range of immune responses and of graft rejection, several groups have selectively bred swine. Now lines of SLA homozygous animals are available for genetic studies of disease resistance and of transplantation responses, as well as for adoptive cell transfers (8, 40-42). The SLA inbred NIH minipigs developed in the U.S. by Sachs and his colleagues are among the best characterized. Derived from one set of parents, they now include 3 homozygous lines of pigs bearing independent SLA haplotypes, designated SLA$^{a/a}$ (aa), cc and dd pigs. In addition SLA recombinants have been found in progeny resulting from cross breedings (10, 43). Established SLA haplotypes of NIH minipigs are demonstrated in Figure 1; in addition, two new SLA recombinants are in the process of being characterized (E. Kortz et al., personal communication).

B. MAb REACTIVE WITH CLASS I SLA ANTIGENS

MAb reactive with class I SLA antigens are listed in Table 1. The top half of the table lists mAb that react with polymorphic determinants of SLA class I antigens, as defined by their differential reactivity on cells from SLA inbred miniature swine of dd, cc, gg, and aa haplotypes and from outbred swine. The bottom half of the table lists mAb that react with monomorphic determinants of class I antigens. In some cases these mAb were tested on mouse L cell lines that had been transfected with, and shown to express,

TABLE 1

mAb Reactive with SLA Class I Antigens

mAb	Ig Class	Alloantigen reactivity[a] dd	cc	gg	aa	Outbred	SLA transfected cells[b] PD1	PD14	Biochemistry[c] Antigen mw (x10³)	First Defined in species[d]	Reference
A. Polymorphic Reactivity											
74-11-10	IgG2b	+	+	+	+	P	+	+	45,12	swine	44
2.2.13	IgM	+	±	±	+	P	-	+	45,12	swine	45
2.12.3	IgM	+	-	-	-	P	-	+	45,12	swine	45
2.28.1	IgM	+	+	+	+	P	+	-		swine	45
2.32.1	IgG	+	-	-	-	P	-	+		swine	45
4.1.56	IgM	+	-	-	+	NT	-	-		swine	45
16.7D4	IgG1	-	+	+	+	NT	-	-		swine	46
16.7E4	IgG1	-	-	-	-	NT	-	-		swine	46
H21A	IgM	-	-	-	-	P	NT			bovine	47, 48
CA48B-A	IgM	+	+	±	+	P	NT			mouse	47, 48
CA4C-A	IgM	+	±	±	+	P	NT			mouse	47, 48
H11A	IgG2a	+	+	+	+	P	NT			bovine	47, 48
H58A	IgG2a	+	-	-	-	P	NT		45,12	bovine	47, 48
H17A	IgG2	-	NT	-	NT	P	NT			bovine	47, 48
H22A	IgG2a	NT	NT	+	+	P	NT			horse	47, 48
3A6		+	±	±	+	NT	NT		45,12	human	49
B. Monomorphic Reactivity											
PT85	IgG2a	+	+	+	+	+	+	+	45,12	bovine	47, 48
2.4.11	IgG1	+	+	+	+	+	+	+	45,12	swine	45
2.13.3	IgG	+	NT	NT	NT	NT	NT		45	swine	45
2.27.3	IgG	+	+	+	+	+	+	+	45,12	swine	45
16.10B4	IgG1	+	+	+	+	+	+	+		swine	46
16.12G8	IgM	+	+	+	+	+	+	-		swine	46
FMD2	IgG2b	NT	NT	NT	NT	+	NT		44,12	swine	50
IIB2	IgG2a	NT	NT	NT	NT	+	NT		44,12	bovine	50
7-34-1	IgG2a	+	+	+	+	+	-	-	45,12	swine	51
3B3		+	+	+	+	+	NT			human	49
9455SA		+	+	+	+	+	NT		45,12	human	e
D4.37HL252		+	+	+	+	+	NT			rat	52
76-7-4	IgG	+	+	+	+	+	NT		40,12	swine	44

[a] mAb reactivity was assessed by mAb mediated cytotoxicity assay, by cell ELISA assay, or by flow cytometric analysis on PBMC from SLA inbred miniature swine or from outbred swine. Reactivity with outbred swine is designated as polymorphic (P) or monomorphic (+).

[b] L cells that have been shown to express the PD1 or PD14 class I SLA gene products, produced by D. Singer et al. (32), were assayed as described above for mAb binding.

[c] Radiolabeled extracts of swine cells were immune precipitated with the mAb noted, facilitated with protein A bearing S. aureus bacteria with or without anti-mouse immunoglobulin. The eluted antigens were analyzed on SDS polyacrylamide gel electrophoresis and molecular weight determined in relation to known standards.

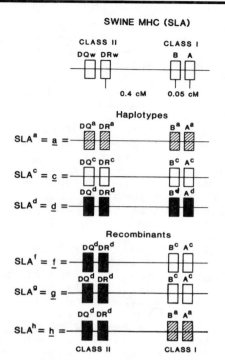

Figure 1.   SLA haplotypes of NIH minipigs

either the PD1 or PD14 SLA class I gene products
(32).   For mAb that react with dd cells this enables
us to assign minimum class I locus reactivity.
However, because the other class I genes have not yet
been successfully expressed in transfected cells, the
total number of class I gene products recognized in
the SLA^d haplotype cannot be accurately assessed.
Moreover, since some of these genes might code for SLA
class I-like differentiation antigens, cells other
than fibroblasts may be required for successful gene
expression.   For other haplotypes L cells expressing
specific class I genes are not available so gene
recognition can only be determined by immunochemical
methods, e.g., sequential immunoprecipitation,
isoelectric focusing or lysostrip analyses.

The mAb that react with monomorphic determinants
of SLA class I genes can be divided into several
groups (Table 1B).   There are those such as PT85 that
react with all cells of every pig tested and with the
two SLA transfected L cells.   These mAb probably
recognize a monomorphic determinant of all classical
SLA class I genes.   Other mAb, like 16.12G8, react

with cells from every pig tested yet only react with
PD1 transfected L cells, indicating it may be
recognizing a monomorphic determinant of possibly a
single genetic locus (46). If it is shown that this
mAb is unreactive with the products of the other SLA
class I genes, then it could be very useful for
determining the locus reactivity of other antibodies,
by using binding inhibition, lysostrip analysis,
and/or immunochemical methods. Thus, even though a
test antibody might not bind to dd PBMC (and therefore
not to L cells that were transfected with dd SLA class
I genes), one could still verify that the antibody
bound to the same locus product on other SLA haplotype
cells using this locus-specific, monomorphic mAb. It
is interesting to note that we have produced several
mAb that react with a monomorphic determinant of the
PD1 gene product but none yet that recognizes a
monomorphic determinant of the PD14 gene product. A
third type of mAb recognizing monomorphic determinants
of SLA class I genes is exemplified by mAb 7-34-1.
This mAb reacts with cells of all pigs and
precipitates a class I type molecule, yet is
unreactive with SLA transfected L cells (51). This
might be a mAb to swine β_2-microglobulin, the
light chain of the SLA class I antigen, which would
not be produced by the mouse L cells. It is equally
likely, that 7-34-1 could be reactive with a
monomorphic determinant of another SLA class I gene
that has not yet been expressed on transfected cells.
At least one cross reactive anti-β_2-microglobulin
has been reported by Teillaud et al. (53). One other
mAb, 76-7-4, which precipitates a class I like protein
of 40,000 and 12,000d MW and reacts with thymocytes,
Langerhans cells and a subset of peripheral blood B
cells, may recognize the pig CD1 molecule or mouse Tla
equivalent (44, Pescovitz et al., manuscript in
preparation).

    MAb reactive with polymorphic SLA class I antigens
can also be divided into several groups distinguished
by their reactivity on cells from the SLA inbred NIH
minipigs and from outbred pigs, by their reactivity on
the L cell transfectants, and by the MW of the antigen
precipitated (Table 1A). Some mAb e.g., 74-11-10,
react with polymorphic determinants of SLA class I
antigens but also recognize the gene products of at
least two separate class I genes, PD1 and PD14 (44,
32). Sequential gel precipitation analysis using this
mAb and alloantibodies that have been selected to
react with only one locus product confirm this
multilocus reactivity (Lunney et al., unpublished

data). There are other mAb, e.g., 2.12.3 and 2.32.1, that react with polymorphic determinants of class I antigens and recognize the PD14 but not the PD1 gene product (45). If either or both of these mAb recognize a unique determinant of the PD14 gene product, they would represent the first mAb reactive with a private SLA specificity. Two other mAb, 16.7D4 and 16.7E4, exhibited differential reactivity, binding cc and gg but not aa or dd PBMC, suggesting that they recognize polymorphic determinants of SLA^c class I antigens. Because they are unreactive with dd PBMC, these mAb are also unreactive with the SLA^d $\overline{DNA}$ derived, PD1 and PD14 L cell transfectants and thus locus reactivity has not yet been mapped. One mAb, 4.1.56, reacts with dd and aa cells but not cc or gg cells. The comparison of dd versus gg and cc links this antigen to the SLA class I genes. If immunoprecipitation studies successfully reveal a class I-like molecule, 4.1.56 could recognize a Qa-like swine cell surface antigen since this mAb recognizes only 50% of PBMC (45). Further tests are needed to verify this hypothesis.

In recent years many laboratories have tried to produce mAb reagents for MHC antigens with the greatest effort being directed towards identifying the human MHC or HLA antigens and the mouse H-2 antigens. Panels of mAb reactive with HLA class I and II antigens have been produced against a wide range of polymorphic, but rarely allelic, specificities as was reported at the HLA Histocompatibility workshop (54, 55). When mice are immunized with cells or with purified antigens from a different species, or even with transfected mouse cells expressing DNA from a foreign species, the resultant antibodies usually recognize common or monomorphic determinants of the foreign species antigens. In fact, if whole peripheral blood mononuclear cells (PBMC) are used as the immunogens, the most likely mAb produced will be those recognizing common lymphoid cell antigens, e.g., the CD4 or CD8 antigens of T cells, or a common, "public" epitope of MHC antigens. Only a subset of mouse mAb to foreign cells will be reactive with polymorphic determinants of the MHC molecules and most of these will be reactive with broadly polymorphic, "public" epitopes of MHC molecules. MAb recognizing unique allelic, "private" polymorphic determinants of the MHC antigens are produced on rare occasions. Almost all of the anti-SLA mAb shown in Table I recognize common monomorphic or "public" polymorphic specificities of SLA class I antigens. To be truly

useful as genetic typing reagents, mAb to MHC antigens
must react only with one unique allele at one genetic
locus, i.e., with a "private" MHC specificity. Such
"private" binding specificity has only been proven by
testing new mAb on a full panel of swine cells that
have previously been proven to express a wide range of
SLA specificities. The new mAb from our laboratory
have been sent to France, Switzerland and Illinois to
test whether they are indeed reactive with any unique
SLA specificities. MAb that react with several
different alleles, i.e., that recognize polymorphic
"public" MHC specificities, are less useful because
both their exact locus reactivity and their allelic
reactions on cells of a new, uncharacterized
individual cannot be predicted.

To overcome the problems associated with rodent
immunizations many laboratories have initiated
production of interspecies hybridomas. Because the
donor cannot make Ab against the common species
antigenic epitopes, fusions using cells from
alloimmunized donors will likely result in the
production of hybridomas secreting mAb reactive with
both public and private polymorphic determinants of
cell surface proteins many of which would be the MHC
antigens because of their strong immunogenicity. The
major drawback of the interspecies hybridomas is their
instability. These hybridomas often lose donor
chromosomes and become unable to secrete mAb.
Moreover, a stable hybridoma cell line may be produced
only after 10-12 subclonings and even then may be
sensitive to the stresses involved in freezing and
thawing (56-59). Thus, even though the expected
results of such interspecies fusions are so desirable
for the goal of obtaining mAb recognizing allelic,
private specificities of SLA antigens, the labor
involved is quite significant. Only two stable
porcine x mouse interspecies hybridomas have been
reported one reactive with an E. coli antigen and the
second against human carcinoembryonic antigen (60,
61). To date, there is no report of an anti-SLA mAb
producing pig x mouse hybridoma cell line.

In summary, a growing panel of mAb reactive with
class I SLA antigens have been developed. Most mAb
were produced by immunization against swine antigens
and appear to react with either monomorphic
determinants or broadly polymorphic "public"
determinants of one or more SLA class I gene
products. However, a few mAb have been identified
that exhibit more restricted reactivity and may be

recognizing unique, "private" SLA class I
specificities.

C.   MAb REACTIVE WITH CLASS II SLA ANTIGENS

MAb reactive with swine class II MHC antigens are
listed in Table 2. When class II SLA specific mAb
were analyzed for polymorphic reactivity, almost none
exhibited differential reactions on cells from SLA
inbred swine. The only mAb that appeared to
recognize polymorphic determinants were 9B, 227 and
Genox 3.53. Each of these mAb appears to have a low
affinity interaction with swine class II antigens, as
indicated by their significantly decreased titers
against swine cells compared to cells of the original
species and by their inability to precipitate class II
glycoproteins from extracts of cells that bound the
mAb. Therefore, they are not very useful for most
analyses (62, Lunney et al., unpublished data). No
mAb to allelic, or even to polymorphic, determinants
of SLA class II antigens appear to have been produced
by any of several fusions using cells from mice
immunized with pig cells (44, 47, 51, 63). In fact,
only one monomorphic anti-SLA class II mAb, MSA3, has
been produced from such a fusion (64). All other
anti-SLA class II mAb are cross reactive mAb that have
been obtained from mice immunized with mouse, bovine
or human cells as noted in Table II.

Since swine class II antigens have recently been
cloned, L-cell transfectants expressing sets of gene
products are just now becoming available for
identifying locus specificity (37). However, unlike
SLA class I proteins for which no MW or significant
isoelectric point differences are evident, the swine
class II gene products have both minor MW and major
isoelectric point differences (24, 38). In addition,
the MW differences of class II, or Ia antigens, are
enhanced under nonreducing conditions. Based on
immunochemical reactivity with extracts of cells
bearing one homozygous SLA haplotype, dd PBMC, MSA-3
and mAb produced against mouse I-E antigens or against
their human equivalent HLA-DR antigens, all reacted
with the SLA-DRw antigens whereas mAb produced against
bovine antigens appeared to recognize SLA-DQw antigens
(24, 38).

Because of their homology with HLA-DR antigens and
with the mouse I-E antigens, the swine Ia antigen
subset precipitated by anti-I-E mAb will be designated
SLA-DRw. The other dominant, lower MW set of swine

TABLE 2

mAb Reactive with SLA class II Antigens

mAb	Ig Class	Characterization of Specificity								First Defined in species[c]	Reference
		Alloantigen Recognition[a]					Biochemistry[b] Antigen MW ($\times 10^{-3}$)				
		dd	cc	gg	aa	Outbred					
SLA-DRw Reactivity											
MSA3	IgG2b, k	+	+	+	+	+	35,28			swine	64
ISCR3	IgG2b, k	+	+	+	+	+	35,28			mouse	65
40B	IgG2a, k	+	+	+	+	+	35,28			mouse	24
9B	IgG2a, k	+	+	−	+	NT[d]	−			mouse	24
40E	IgG2a, k	+	+	+	+	NT	35,28			mouse	24
39D	IgG2a, k	+	+	+	+	NT	35,28			mouse	24
40K	IgG2a, k	+	+	+	+	NT	35,28			mouse	24
39G	IgG2a, k	+	+	+	+	NT	35,28			mouse	24
40D	IgG2a, k	+	+	+	+	+	35,28			mouse	24
7A	IgG2a, k	+	+	+	+	+	35,28			mouse	24
74C	IgG3, k	+	+	+	+	+	35,28			mouse	24
DC2.06	IgG2	+	+	+	+	+	35,28			human	66
SLA-DQw Reactivity											
TH16B	IgG2a, k	+	+	+	+	+	34,27			bovine	47,48
H42A	IgG2a, k	+	+	+	+	+	34,27			bovine	47,48
TH21A	IgG2a, k	+	+	+	+	+	34,27			bovine	47,48
TH22	IgG2a, k	+	+	+	+	+	34,27			bovine	47,48
RH1A	IgG2a, k	+	+	+	+	+	34,27			bovine	47,48
SLA Class II Reactivity											
227		−	−	NT	+	NT	−			human	62
Genox 3.53	IgG3	+	−	NT	+	NT	−			human	62
H4		NT	+	NT	NT	+	NT			human	67
TH4B		+	+	NT	+	+	NT			bovine	47,48
TH14B	IgM	NT	NT	NT	NT	+	NT			bovine	47,48
TH81B		NT	NT	NT	NT	+	NT			bovine	47,48

[a] Analyses performed as described in legend 1 of Table 1.

[b] Analyses performed as described in legend 3, Table 1, except all gels run under non-reducing conditions. A dash denotes no immunoprecipitation with a given mAb though other mAb were positive on the same gel.

[c] Reactivity of some mAb was first characterized on the species shown and then they were used to analyze swine class II antigens.

class II antigens will be designated the SLA-DQw antigens in analogy to HLA-DQ antigens. Recent flow cytometric analyses of L cell transfectants revealed that 40D and ISCR3 reacted only with L cells transfected with SLA-DR alpha and beta chains whereas TH16 and TH22 reacted only with SLA-DQ alpha and beta chains (F. Hirsch et al., unpublished data). These results confirm the SLA locus assignment of mAb reactivity. The SLA-DRw and SLA-DQw subsets of swine class II antigens have also been demonstrated to be independent sets of antigens on dd PBMC by sequential immunoprecipitation analysis using mAb 40D and TH16 (38, Lunney et al., unpublished data). SLA-DPw proteins may be included in the Ia antigens precipitated in these gels, but antibodies that react exclusively with this subset of swine class II antigens have not yet been identified, nor has it been confirmed that the putative SLA-DP genes exist or are transcribed into surface proteins. Future DNA and cell transfection experiments will help define the true genetic complexity of the SLA-D region, including the numbers of expressed α and β genes for each locus.

It is intriguing to speculate why there are so few anti-SLA class II mAb produced from mice immunized with pig cells. One might expect that because of the interspecies class II antigen cross reactions that the SLA class II antigens would be less immunogenic. However, the one mAb, MSA3, produced from mice immunized with Concanavalin A activated pig PBMC (64) reacts with SLA-DRw antigens, the same subset of class II antigens that are recognized by the cross reactive anti-mouse I-E mAb. It is the second class II antigen subset, the mouse I-A or swine SLA-DQw antigens, for which mAb have only been produced in mice immunized with cells of different livestock species (38, 47). It is possible that bovine and equine cells express more of the DQ antigens. However, not only do swine have normal B cell and macrophage expression of class II antigens but they also express class II antigens on a significant percentage of T cells, particularly the CD8[+] subset; the SLA-DQw antigens are expressed at lower levels than the SLA-DRw antigens on this T cell subset (39). Our recent interspecies hybridoma fusions may have produced some anti-class II mAb; we are currently cloning, freezing and characterizing their supernatant mAb (Sun et al., unpublished data). In summary, there is no obvious reason why more hybridomas secreting mAb specific for pig class II antigens have not been produced from

direct fusions of cells from mice immunized with pig
cells. Con A or γ-interferon stimulation of pig
PBMC should lead to expression of higher levels of SLA
class II antigens, thus, immunization with such
stimulated cells may help to overcome this problem.

The interspecies anti-class II mAb cross reactions
reveal potential evolutionary relationships between
class II antigens. The cross reaction of anti-mouse
class II Ab on cells from humans and pigs down to
chicken and frog highlighted the evolutionary
relatedness of the SLA-DR equivalent antigens in these
species (68). Mouse anti-I-E alloantisera are
reactive with bovine cells (69). However in recent
studies we have determined that some of the cross
reactive anti-I-E mAb do not react with bovine or
ovine cells (Lunney et al., unpublished data), Thus,
there may be a limitation on the epitopes of the DR
subset of antigens that cross reactive mAb recognize.
Moreover, several species, such as cow, sheep and
horses, share extensive DQ subset class II antigen
cross reactions with the pig as determined by mAb
binding. This reactivity may be shared as well with
human and rodent antigens, although the locus
reactivity of each of these cross reactive mAb has not
yet been determined for each species (47, 48).
Further exploration of these relationships using cells
that express cloned genes and comparing sequences of
these genes should help to delineate the exact
evolutionary relationship among these genes.

Most of the mAb listed in Table II react with
monomorphic determinants of class II antigens and
therefore have limited applicability in functional
assays. Detailed analysis of monomorphic anti-human
class II MHC mAb has revealed that some mAb appeared
to react with monomorphic determinants of one locus.
In certain haplotypes, however, these same mAb
cross-recognized an allelic determinant of a second
locus product (70). Many other types of cross
reactions between class II products were found by
these authors and by others (54, 55). Thus, if one
wants to use mAb to assign certain functions to
specific gene products, one must know the exact locus
reactivity of each mAb on cells of each haplotype to
be tested, e.g., a mAb may recognize the SLA-DQ
antigens expressed by every pig cell and, in addition,
recognize an allelic product of one SLA-DR gene that
is expressed on cells of a single haplotype such as
SLA^d.

In summary, antigens encoded by at least two separate SLA-D region loci have been identified and characterized using several different mAb reactive mainly with monomorphic determinants of each locus product. The positive mAb were generally produced in immunizations against other species and later identified as cross-reactive with swine class II antigens. MAb that recognize unique, polymorphic determinants of swine Ia antigens await future fusions using purified antigens, such as have been performed by Barber and his colleagues (71, and personal communication), or new SLA-D gene transfectants as immunogens. Alternatively, the generation of a swine myeloma fusion partner would enable us to produce swine anti-swine mAb.

D.   USE OF MAb TO ANALYZE SLA GENE EXPRESSION AND FUNCTION

Baseline parameters of SLA class I and II distribution on important lymphoid cell populations must be established before questions of SLA function can be addressed in in vitro assays. All mature lymphocytes express high levels of class I antigens whereas there is a differential expression of class II antigens. As expected, B cells and macrophages express both SLA-DRw and DQw antigens but, unexpectedly, T cells express higher levels of SLA-DRw than DQw antigens (26, 39). Unlike guinea pigs, dogs and cattle where all T cells express class II antigens, and most other species where T cells are class II negative; in swine there is preferential expression of class II antigens on the CD8$^+$ T cell subset (26, Pescovitz et al., manuscript in preparation). The importance/relevance of this unusual class II T cell expression has yet to be fully explored.

In fact, assessment of normal SLA gene expression is only a basis for other studies on the modulation of SLA antigen expression and on the resultant stimulation or suppression of immune responses that occur during immune or disease responses. Since γ-interferon clearly enhances SLA class I expression (72) and is produced during viral infection, this would be only one potential mode of changing immune responses. Our earlier work also showed that class II expression on PBMC is enhanced during an active Ascaris suum infection (73). One method of determining the functional significance of SLA gene products is establishing in vitro assays which reflect

in vivo immune responses and using anti-SLA mAb to
block the relevant cellular interactions.

Class II SLA antigens were originally defined by
cellular mixed lymphocyte reactivity, or MLR (8), the
proliferation that results when responder cells that
express class II antigens of one set of SLA
haplotype(s) are cocultured with stimulator cells
bearing a different set of SLA haplotypes(s).   In
preliminary studies using mAb to monomorphic class II
determinants, anti-SLA-DQw mAb easily blocked swine
MLR blastogenesis (38, Lunney et al., manuscript in
preparation). Depletion of responder cells of all
class II positive cells resulted in a predominantly
CD4$^+$ class II$^-$ T cell preparation whose MLR
induced blastogenesis was easily blocked by
anti-SLA-DQw mAb and, at higher levels, by
anti-SLA-DRw mAb. This indicates that in the pig both
SLA-DRw and -DQw loci may be important for the
propagation of the MLR responses, as has been found in
certain haplotype combinations in human MLR responses
(74). Testing mAb that recognize allelic determinants
of SLA antigens will facilitate these studies by
allowing dissection of the effects of stimulator from
responder cell surface molecules.

Collaborative studies with scientists at the Plum
Island Animal Disease Center using cells from animals
who recovered from African swine fever virus (ASFV)
infections have demonstrated virus specific cytotoxic
and proliferative T cell responses including
stimulation of production of high levels of
interleukin-2 (75, 76). The virus specific cytotoxic
cells have been shown to be SLA class I restricted by
blocking with anti-SLA class I specific mAb and by
depletion of killer cells with anti-CD8 mAb (75).
Future adoptive cell transfer studies will determine
whether either these CD8$^+$ SLA class I restricted
cytotoxic T cells or potential CD4$^+$ class II
restricted blastogenic cells induce a protective
immune response against this lethal virus infection in
naive pigs.

These ASFV restricted T cell responses are further
complicated by the modulation of expression of swine
MHC class I and class II antigens in cells of the
mononuclear phagocytic system during infection with
ASFV. At 12 hr post-infection, ASFV infected
macrophages had a significant decrease in SLA class I
antigens while class II expression was not impaired
(M. Gonzalez-Juarrero et al., manuscript in

preparation). These results and analyses of cryostat sections from ASFV infected tissues clearly indicated that modulations in the expression of SLA antigens occurred during ASFV infection. Further functional studies must be done to determine if these modulations in MHC antigen expression influence humoral and cellular immune response in ASFV infection.

In summary, these few examples from our own research of uses of mAb to SLA class I and II antigens to assess gene expression and function barely begin to highlight the importance of SLA antigens in regulating basic swine immune responses. Future research will undoubtedly prove that SLA class I and II antigens are intimately involved in many disease responses and in determining vaccine effectiveness. Development of panels of SLA class I and II reactive mAb will serve to accelerate such progress and enhance our understanding of factors that regulate swine immune responses.

Acknowledgments

We thank Drs. Hyun Lillehoj, Thor Sundt and Mark Failla for their critical reviews of this manuscript. D. Ivanoska was supported in part by USDA, OICD, Agricultural Scholarship Program for Middle Income Countries and D. Sun by USDA, CSRS grant #85-CRCR-1-1708. W. C. Davis is supported by USDA, SEA grants 83 CRSR-2-2281, 86 CRSR-2-2913, and 86 CRCR-1-2241, by WSU-ARC 3073, by formula funding Public Law 95-113 and by Washington State Technology Center.

References:

1. Grumet, F.C., G.F. Mitchell and H.O. McDevitt. 1971. Genetic control of specific immune responses in inbred mice. Ann. NY Acad. Sci. 190:170-177.
2. Schwartz, R.H. 1986. Immune response (Ir) genes of the murine major histocompatibility complex. Adv. Immunol. 38:31-201.
3. Herrington, D.A., D.F. Clyde, G. Losonsky, M. Cortesia, J.R. Murphy, J. Davis, S. Baqar, A.M. Felix, F.P. Heimer, D. Gillessen, V. Nussensweig, M.R. Hollingdale and M.M. Levine. 1987. Safety and immunogenicity in man of a synthetic peptide malaria vaccine against Plasmodium falciparum sporozoites. Nature 328:257-259.

4. Good, M.F., J.A. Berzofsky, W.L. Maloy, Y.
    Hayashi, N. Fujii, W.T. Hockmeyer, and L.H.
    Miller. 1986. Genetic control of the immune
    response in mice to a Plasmodium falciparum
    sporozoite vaccine: Widespread
    non-responsiveness to single malaria T epitope in
    highly repetitive vaccine. J. Exper. Med.
    164:655-660.

5. Hoffman, S.L., L.T. Cannon, Sr., J.A. Berzofsky,
    W.R. Majarian, J.F. Young, W.L. Meloy, and W.T.
    Hockmeyer. 1987. Plasmodium falciparum.
    Sporozoite boosting of immunity due to a T-cell
    epitope on a sporozoite vaccine. Exper.
    Parasitol. 64:64-70.

6. Nishimoti, H., H. Kikutani, K. Yamamura, T.
    Kishimoto. 1987. Prevention of autoimmune
    insulitis by expression of I-E molecule in NOD
    mice. Nature 328:432-433.

7. Vaiman, M., C. Renard, P. Lafage, J. Ametean and
    P. Nizza. 1970. Evidence for a histocompati-
    bility system in swine (SL-A). Transplantation
    10:155-164.

8. Viza, D., J.R. Sugar, and R.M. Binns. 1970.
    Lymphocyte stimulation in pigs. Evidence for the
    existence of a single major histocompatibility
    locus: PL-A. Nature 227:949-951.

9. Vaiman, M., J. Metzger, C. Renard and J. Vila.
    1978. Immune response gene(s) controlling the
    humoral anti-lysozyme response (Ir-Lys) linked to
    the major histocompatibility complex SL-A in the
    pig. Immunogenetics 7:231-243.

10. Lunney, J.K., M.D. Pescovitz, and D.H. Sachs.
    1986a. The swine major histocompatibility
    complex: Its structure and function. In: M.E.
    Tumbleson (Ed.). Swine in Biomedical Research.
    New York: Plenum Press, pp. 1821-1836.

11. Rothschild, M.F., H.L. Chen, L.L. Christian, W.R.
    Lie, L. Venier, M. Cooper, C. Briggs and C.M.
    Warner. 1984a. Breed and swine lymphocyte
    antigen haplotype differences in agglutination
    titers following vaccination with
    B. Bronchiseptica. J. Animal Sci. 59:643-649.

12. Rothschild, M.F., H.T. Hill, L. L. Christian and
    C.M. Warner. 1984b. Genetic differences in
    serum neutralization titers of pigs after
    vaccination with pseudorabies modified live-virus
    vaccine. Am J. Vet. Res. 45:1216-1218.

13. Lunney, J.K. and K.D. Murrell. 1988.
    Immunogenetic analysis of Trichinella spiralis
    infections in swine. Veterinary Parasitology, in
    press.

14. Madden, K.B., K.D. Murrell, and J.K. Lunney.
     1988. Elimination of mature encapsulated
     <u>Trichinella</u> <u>spiralis</u> muscle larvae after
     secondary infection of SLA$^{a/a}$ miniature swine.
     FASEB J. 2:A680.

15. Capy, P., C. Renard, P. Sellier, and M. Vaiman.
     1981. Etude preliminaire des relations entre le
     complex majeur d'histocompatibilities (SLA) et
     des caracteres de production chez le Porc. Ann.
     Genet. Sel. Anim. 13:441-446.

16. Rothschild, M.F., D.R. Zimmerman, R.K. Johnson,
     L. Venier and C.M. Warner. 1985. SLA haplotype
     differences in lines of pigs which differ in
     ovulation rate. Animal Blood Groups and
     Biochemical Genetics. 15:155-158.

17. Rothschild, M.F., C. Renard, G. Bolet, P. Dando
     and M. Vaiman. 1986. Effects of swine
     lymphocyte antigen haplotype on birth and weaning
     weights in pigs. Anim. Genet. 17:267-272.

18. Mallard, B.A., B.N. Wilkie, B.A. Croy, B.W.
     Kennedy, and R. Friendship. 1987. Influence of
     the swine major histocompatibility complex on
     reproductive traits in miniature swine. J.
     Reprod. Immunol. 12:201-214.

19. Vaiman, M., C. Renard, and N. Bourgeaux. 1988.
     The SLA complex, the major histocompatibility
     system in swine: Its influence on physiological
     and pathological traits. In C. Warner, M.
     Rothschild and S. Lamont (Eds.). The molecular
     biology of the major histocompatibility complex
     of domestic animal species. Ames, Iowa: ISU
     Press. In press.

20. Vaiman, M., P. Chardon, and C. Renard. 1979.
     Genetic organization of one pig SLA complex.
     Studies on nine recombinants and biochemical and
     lysostrip analysis. Immunogenetics 9:353-362.

21. Lunney, J.K., and D.H. Sachs. 1978.
     Transplantation in miniature swine. IV.
     Chemical characterization of MSLA and Ia-like
     antigens. J. Immunol. 120:607-612.

22. Soloski, M., J. Vernachio, G. Einhorn and A.
     Lattimore. 1986. Qa gene expression:
     Biosynthesis and secretion of Qa-2 molecules in
     activated T cells. Proc. Natl. Acad. Sci.
     83:2949-2953.

23. Chardon, P., C. Renard and M. Vaiman. 1981.
     Characterization of class II histocompatibility
     antigens in pigs. An. Blood Groups Biochem Gen.
     12:59-65.

24. Lunney, J.K., B.A. Osborne, S.O. Sharrow, C. Devaux, M. Pierres, and D.H. Sachs. 1983. Sharing of Ia antigens between species. IV. Interspecies cross-reactivity of monoclonal antibodies directed against polymorphic mouse Ia determinants. J. Immunol. 130:2786-2793.
25. Thistlethwaite, J.R., L.R. Pennington, J.K. Lunney, and D.H. Sachs. 1983. Immunologic characterization of MHC recombinant swine. Production of SLA class specific antisera and detection of Ia antigens on both B and non-B PBL. Transplantation 35:394-400.
26. Pescovitz, M.D., F. Popitz, D.H. Sachs and J.K. Lunney. 1985. Expression of Ia antigens on resting porcine T cells. A marker of functional T cells subsets. In Streilein, J.W. et al. (Eds.). Advances in Gene Technology: Molecular Biology of the Immune System. ICSU Press. p. 271-272.
27. Lunney, J.K., and Pescovitz, M.D. 1988. Differentiation antigens of swine lymphoid tissues. In Trnka, Z., and Miyasaka, M. (Eds.). Comparative Aspects of Differentiation Antigens. New York: Marcel Dekkar, Inc., pp. 421-454.
28. Albert, E.D., M.P. Baur and W.R. Mayr. 1985. Histocompatibility Testing, 1984. New York: Springer-Verlag.
29. Kindt, T.J., and M.A. Robinson. 1984. Major histocompatibility complex antigens. In W.E. Paul (Ed.). Fundamental Immunology, New York: Raven Press, pp 347-378.
30. Klein, J. 1986. Natural History of the Major Histocompatibility Complex. New York: J. Wiley and Sons.
31. Singer, D.S., R.D. Camerini-Otero, M.L. Satz, B. Osborne, D. Sachs, and S. Rudikoff. 1982. Characterization of a porcine genomic clone encoding a major histocompatibility antigen: Expression in mouse L cells. Proc Natl. Acad. Sci. USA 79:1403-1407.
32. Singer, D.S., R. Ehrlich, H. Golding, L. Satz, L. Parent, and S. Rudikoff. 1988. Structure and expression of class I MHC genes in the miniature swine. In: C. Warner, M. Rothschild, and S. Lamont (Eds.): The Molecular Biology of the Major Histocompatibility Complex of Domestic Animal Species. Ames, IA: ISU Press. In press.

33. Chardon P., C. Renard, M. Kirszenbaum, C. Geffrotin, D. Cohen, and M. Vaiman. 1985a. Molecular genetic analysis of the major histocompatibility complex in pig families and recombinants. J. Immunogenet. 12:139-149.

34. Chardon, P., M. Vaiman, M. Kirszenbaum, C. Geffrotin, C. Renard, and D. Cohen. 1985b. Restriction fragment length polymorphism of the major histocompatibility complex of the pig. Immunogenetics 21:161-171.

35. Ehrlich, R., R. Lifshitz, M.D. Pescovitz, S. Rudikoff, and D.S. Singer. 1987. Tissue specific expression and structure of a divergent member of a class I MHC gene family. J. Immunol. 139:593-602.

36. Warner, C.M. 1986. Genetic manipulation of the major histocompatibility complex. J. Anim. Sci. 63:279-287.

37. Sachs, D.H., S. Germana, M. El-Gamil, K. Gustafsson, F. Hirsch and K. Pratt. 1988. Class II genes of miniature swine. I. Class II gene characterization by RFLP and by isolation from a genomic library. Immunogenetics. In press.

38. Lunney, J.K., W.C. Davis, and M.D. Pescovitz. 1985. Identification of monoclonal antibodies that recognize the SLA-DwQ antigens, a second set of swine Ia antigens. Fed. Proc. 44:554.

39. Lunney, J.K., and M.D. Pescovitz. 1987. Phenotypic and functional characterization of pig lymphocyte populations. Vet. Immunol. Immunopath. 17:135-144.

40. Sachs, D.H., G. Leight, J. Cone, S. Schwartz, L. Stuart and S. Rosenberg. 1976. Transplantation in miniature swine. I. Fixation of the major histocompatibility complex. Transplant. 22:559-567.

41. Binns, R.M., and S.T. Licence. 1983. Long term survival of MHC-compatible lymphocytes and two phase clearance of allogeneic incompatible lymphocytes in the young pig. Immunol. 49:727-731.

42. Hradecky, J., V. Hruban, J. Hojny, J. Pazdera, and R. Stanck. 1985. Development of a semi-inbred line of Landrace pigs. I. Breeding performance and immunogenetic characteristics. Lab. Anim. 19:279-283.

43. Pennington, L.R., J.K. Lunney and D.H. Sachs. 1981. Transplantation in miniature swine. VIII. Recombination within the MHC of miniature swine. Transplantation 31:66-72.

44.   Pescovitz, M.D., J.K. Lunney and D.H. Sachs.
      1984.   Preparation and characterization of
      monoclonal antibodies reactive with PBL.   J.
      Immunol. 133:368-375.
45.   Ivanoska, D., D.C. Sun, and J.K. Lunney.   1988.
      Production of monoclonal antibodies reactive with
      polymorphic and monomorphic determinants of SLA
      class I gene products.   Manuscript submitted.
46.   Sun, D.C., B.E. Atkin, and J.K. Lunney.   1988.
      Production and characterization of monoclonal
      antibodies (mAb) reactive with gene products of
      swine major histocompatibility complex (SLA).
      FASEB J. 2:A480.
47.   Davis, W.C., L.E. Perryman, and T.C. McGuire.
      1984.   The identification and analysis of major
      functional populations of differentiated cells.
      In: N.J. Stern, and H.R. Gamble (Eds.):
      Hybridoma Technology in Agricultural and
      Veterinary Research.   Totowa, New Jersey: Rowman
      and Allanheld, pp. 121-150.
48.   Davis, W.C., S. Marusic, H.A. Lewin, G.A.
      Splitter, L.E. Perryman, T.C. McGuire, and J.R.
      Gorham.   1987.   The development and analysis of
      species specific and cross reactive monoclonal
      antibodies to leukocyte differentiation antigens
      and antigens of the major histocompatibility
      complex for use in the study of the immune system
      in cattle and other species.   Vet. Immunol.
      Immunopathol. 15:337-376.
49.   Haynes, B.F., M.E. Hemler, D.L. Mann, G.S.
      Eisenbarth, J. Shelhamer, H.S. Mostowski, C.A.
      Thomas, J.L. Strominger and A.S. Fauci.   1981.
      Characterization of a monoclonal antibody, 4F-2,
      that binds to human monocytes and to a subset of
      activated lymphocytes.   J. Immunol. 126:1409-1414.
50.   Letesson, J.-J., P. Coppe, N. Lostrie, R.
      Creimers and A. Depelchin.   1986.   Production and
      characterization of monoclonal antibodies raised
      against BoLA class I antigens.   Vet. Immunol.
      Immunopathol. 13:213-226.
51.   Lie, W.-R., M.F. Rothschild, and C.M. Warner.
      1986.   Preparation and characterization of
      monoclonal antibodies to swine lymphocyte
      antigens.   Fed. Proc. 45:987.
52.   Smilek, D.E., H.C. Boyd, D.B. Wilson, C.M.
      Zmijewski, F.W. Fitch, and T.J. McKearn.   1980.
      Monoclonal rat anti-major histocompatibility
      complex antibodies display specificity for rat,
      mouse, and human target cells.   J. Exper. Med.
      151:1139-1150.

53. Teillaud, J.-L., D. Crevat, P. Chardon, J. Kalil,
     C. Goujet-Zalc, G. Mahouy, M. Vaiman, M. Fellows,
     and D. Pious. 1982. Monoclonal antibodies as a
     tool for phylogenetic studies of major
     histocompatibility antigens and
     β_2-microglobulins. Immunogenetics 15:377-384.

54. Fauchet, R., J.G. Bodmer, L. J. Kennedy, M.C.
     Mazzilli, C. Müller, C. Raffoux, and P.
     Richiardi. 1984. Joint report: HLA-A, B, C
     monoclonal antibodies. In: E.D. Albert, M.P.
     Baur, and W.R. Mayr (Eds.): Histocompatibility
     Testing 1984. New York: Springer-Verlag,
     pp. 211-217.

55. Bodmer, J.G., L. J. Kennedy, M. Aizawa, R. L.
     Dawkins, V. Lepage, M. C. Mazzilli, and P.
     Richiardi. 1984. HLA-D region monoclonal
     antibodies. In E.D. Albert, M.P. Baur, and W.R.
     Mayr (Eds.) Histocompatibility Testing 1984.
     New York: Springer Verlag, pp. 217-236.

56. Tucker, E.M., A.R. Dain, S.W. Clarke, and R.
     Donker. 1984. Specific bovine monoclonal
     antibody produced by a refused mouse/calf
     hybridoma. Hybridoma. 3:171-176.

57. Anderson, D.V., E.M. Tucker, J.R. Powell, and P.
     Porter. 1987. Bovine monoclonal antibodies to
     the F5 (K99) pilus antigen of E. coli, produced
     by murine/bovine hybridomas. Vet. Immunol.
     Immunopath. 15:223-237.

58. Srikumaran, S., A.J. Guidry, and R.A. Goldsby.
     1983. Bovine x mouse hybridomas that secrete
     bovine immunoglobulin G_1. Science 220:522-523.

59. Srikumaran, S., A.J. Guidry, and R.A. Goldsby.
     1984. Production and characterization of
     monoclonal bovine immunoglobulin G_1, G_2, and
     M from bovine x murine hybridomas. Vet. Immunol.
     Immunopath. 5:323-342.

60. Raybould, T.J.G., P.J. Willson, L.J. McDougall,
     and T.C. Watts. 1985. A porcine-murine
     hybridoma that secretes porcine monoclonal
     antibody of defined specificity. Am. J. Vet.
     Res. 46:1768-1769.

61. Buchegger, F., K. Fournier, M. Schreyer, S.
     Carrel and J.-P. Mach. 1987. Swine monoclonal
     antibodies of high affinity and specificity to
     carcinoembryonic antigen. J. Natl. Cancer Inst.
     79:337-342.

62. Lunney, J.K., B.A. Osborne, J.-J. Metzger, G.L.
     Gilliland, S. Rudikoff, and D.H. Sachs. 1981.
     Reactions of monoclonal antibodies with swine MHC
     antigens. Fed. Proc. 40:1053.

63. Jonjic, S., and Koszinowski, U., 1984.
     Monoclonal antibodies reactive with swine
     lymphocytes I. Antibodies to membrane structures
     that define the cytolytic T lymphocyte subset in
     the swine. J. Immunol. 133:647-652.
64. Hammerburg, C., and G. Schurig. 1986.
     Characterization of monoclonal antibodies
     directed against swine leukocytes. Vet. Immunol.
     Immunopath. 11:107-121.
65. Watanabe, M., T. Suzuki, M. Taniguchi, and N.
     Shinohara. 1983. Monoclonal anti-Ia murine
     alloantibodies crossreactive with the
     Ia-homologues of other mammalian species
     including humans. Transplantation 36:712-716.
66. Osborne, B.A., J.K. Lunney, L.R. Pennington, D.H.
     Sachs, and S. Rudikoff. 1984. Two dimensional
     gel analysis of swine histocompatibility
     antigens. J. Immunol. 131:2939-2944.
67. Lewin, H.A., C.C. Calvert and D. Bernoco. 1985.
     Cross-reactivity of a monoclonal antibody with
     bovine, equine, ovine and porcine peripheral
     blood B lymphocytes. Am. J. Vet. Res. 46:785-788.
68. Shinohara, N. and D.H. Sachs. 1982.
     Interspecies cross reactions of murine anti-Ia
     antibodies. In Ferrone S. and C.S. David
     (Eds.). Ia Antigens. vol. I Mice. Boca Raton,
     FL: CRC Press, Inc., p. 219-240.
69. Hoang-Xuan, M., D. Charron, M.-T. Zilber and D.
     Levy. 1982. Biochemical characterization of
     class II bovine major histocompatibility complex
     antigens using cross-species reactive
     antibodies. Immunogenetics. 15:621-624.
70. Shaw, S., A. Ziegler and R. DeMars. 1985.
     Specificity of monoclonal antibodies directed
     against human and murine class II
     histocompatibility antigens as analyzed by
     binding to HLA-deletion mutant cell lines. Human
     Immunology 12:191-211.
71. Alting-Mees, M., and B.H. Barber. 1986. A
     structural analysis of the carbohydrate side
     chains on class I and class II histocompatibility
     antigens of the swine facilitated by
     heteroantisera specific for the denatured
     polypeptides. Mol. Immunol. 23:847-861.
72. Satz, M.L., and D.S. Singer. 1984. Effect of
     mouse interferon on the expression of a porcine
     major histocompatibility gene introduced into
     mouse L cells. J. Immunol. 132:496-502.

73. Lunney, J.K., J.F. Urban, Jr., and L.A. Johnson.
     1986b. Protective immunity to <u>Ascaris</u> <u>suum</u>:
     analysis of swine peripheral blood cell subsets
     using monoclonal antibodies and flow cytometry.
     Vet. Parasitol. 20:117-131.
74. Eckels, D.D., and A. Zeevi. 1986. Structural
     and functional relationships of human class II
     MHC molecules. Human Immunol. 15:68-74.
75. Martins, C., C. Mebus, T. Scholl, M. Lawman, and
     J. Lunney. 1988. Virus specific CTL in SLA
     inbred swine recovered from experimental African
     swine fever virus infection. Annals NY Acad.
     Sci. In Press.
76. Scholl, T., J.K. Lunney, C.A. Mebus, E. Duffy and
     C.L.V. Martins. 1988. Virus specific cellular
     blastogenesis and Interleukin-2 production in
     African swine fever virus (ASFV) recovered pigs.
     Manuscript submitted.

Cloning of Chicken Major Histocompatibility (B) Complex and T Cell Differentiation Antigen Genes by Using Mammalian DNA Probes: Current Status

8

Ghislaine Béhar, Alain Bernot, Yves Bourlet, François Guillemot, Rima Zoorob, and Charles Auffray

The molecular cloning of chicken MHC and T cell differentiation antigen genes has been approached by using homologous mammalian probes in cross-hybridization experiments. This has allowed isolation of MHC class II (B-L) beta chain sequences sharing at least 61% of their nucleotides with homologous HLA probes. In contrast, human or mouse probes for class II alpha chains, the class II associated invariant chain, class I alpha chains and beta 2-microglobulin, T cell receptor alpha, beta and gamma chains and the associated T3 delta and epsilon chains, and Thy-1 yielded negative results. The B-L probe provides a point of entry to the B complex which can be analyzed by chromosome walking.

Over the past seven years, an overwhelming amount of information has been accumulated on the structure of the major histocompatibility complex of mammals by using recombinant DNA techniques (1,2). The gene products themselves are much better defined and their functional role can be approached by gene transfer techniques in cultured cells or transgenic animals. One of the major goals of these studies is to build a molecular map of the gene complex and to pinpoint the genes that are responsible for the strong linkage observed between various diseases and certain MHC alleles or haplotypes. In this regard the chicken appears as an excellent system since the capacity to develop or regress tumors induced by Rous sarcoma virus is controlled by the major histocompatibility (B) complex, and certain alleles of this complex (B21) confer a high degree of resistance to the development of Marek's disease, a lymphoma induced by a herpes virus (3).

Moreover, the possibility of studying the development of the immune system in ovo makes it an ideal system to approach the problems of thymic

Institut d'Embryologie du CNRS et du Collège de France, 49 bis, avenue de la Bella Gabrielle 94130 Nogent sur Marne, France.

education and tolerance induction during ontogeny, with the prospect of manipulating the various facets of the immune system in an easier way than in rodent embryos. In addition, since birds have evolved separately from mammals for approximately 270 million years, the comparison of the structures (genes and proteins) that control the immune system in these two classes of vertebrates could provide a better understanding of their function at the molecular level. All these considerations also apply to the functional partners of the major histocompatibility complex antigen, the T cell receptor chains and the various accessory molecules expressed at different stages of T cell differentiation.

This requires that the MHC and T cell antigens of the chicken should be described at the protein and gene level in a similar fashion to mammals. When considering the possible approaches to this problem, one has to remember that the human and mouse MHC genes have been isolated using several independent strategies which were all based on the use of antibodies against the polypetide chains either used to immunoprecipitate polysomes or cell-free translation products, or to obtain amino acid sequence information on the purified material and derive from it synthetic oligonucleotide probes. Subsequently, the first isolated probes were used to isolate cross-hybridizing sequences either in the same species or in another mammalian species. The T cell receptor chains have been isolated using potent subtractive or differential hybridization procedures, which select those sequences expressed specifically in T cells and subject to somatic rearrangement (4). The other T cell differentiation antigen genes have been isolated using the same techniques used for the MHC genes or a combination of gene transfer and substractive hybridization procedures. Although these approaches can be repeated to isolate the MHC and T cell specific genes of the chicken, it will require an enormous amount of work. Many of these genes belong to subfamilies of the immunoglobulin gene superfamily and are clustered on a limited number of chromosomes. This is the case of all MHC genes which are located in a single complex. We have approached the molecular characterization of these genes in the chicken by attempting to identify at least one member of each gene complex which can provide a point of entry to obtain the other genes by chromosome walking experiments, and we have first investigated the possibility of using the available mammalian probes in cross-hybridization experiments. Here we report the current status of these experiments.

Materials and Methods

Library screening

Phage clones from chicken genomic and cDNA libraries were plated at 40.000 plaques per 150 mm diameter Petri dish, and transferred to nitrocellulose filters (Millipore HAHY). The filters were prewashed 2 hrs at 42°C in 50mM Tris pH 8.0, 1M NaCl, 1 mM EDTA, 0.1% SDS, and prehybridized 4 hrs at 42°C in 50% formamide, 5x Denhardt, 5x SSPE, 0.1% SDS, 1 ug/ml poly (A), 1 ug/ml poly (C), 100 ug/ml denatured salmon sperm DNA. DNA fragments were isolated by electrophoresis on a 5% polyacrylamide gel by electroelution and DEAE-cellulose chromatography and labeled by nick-translation to a specific activity of $2-4.10^8$ cpm/ug. Hybridization was for 24 hrs at 42°C followed by 24 hrs at 37°C to ensure stabilization of the hybrids. The filters were washed 2x 1 hr at 45°C and 2x 1 hr at 55°C in 2x SSC, 0.1% SDS exposed to Kodak X-OMAT AR5 films for 2-7 days at -80°C with two intensifying screens (Dupont Li Plus).

Northern blot analysis

Poly A^+-RNA was prepared by the LiCl urea method followed by oligo-dT cellulose chromatography, from chicken liver, spleen, thymus, the B cell line RP9 and the T cell line MSB1, as well as control human and mouse tissues : the human B cell line CA, human and mouse thymus, mouse spleen and the mouse B cell line Sp2/0. The Northern blots were prehybridized for 4 hrs at 42°C in 50mM Na Phosphate pH 6.5, 50% formamide, 5x SSC, 1x Denhardt, 250 ug/ml sonicated salmon sperm DNA. Hybridization was in the same buffer at 37°C for 16 hrs with 10^6 cpm/ml of denatured nick-translated probe labeled by nick-translation at a specific activity of $1-4.10^8$ cpm/ug of DNA fragment purified by polyacrylamide gel electrophoresis. Posthybridization washing was performed in 2x SSC, 1% SDS by stepwise temperature increments: 1x 15' at 30°C, 2x 60' at 40°C, 2x 60' at 40°C and optional final washes at 50°C depending on monitored background. The blots were exposed to Kodak X-OMAT AR5 films for 1-7 days at -80°C with intensifying screens.

Results and discussion

Isolation of chicken class II beta chain genes

We first used a SacI-EcoRI DNA fragment derived from an HLA-DQ beta probe to search for homologous sequences by Northern blot analysis in chicken tissues and detected faint signals at the appropriate size (around 1.2-1.3Kb). Subsequently the same probe was used to screen available chicken genomic DNA libraries and several phage clones were obtained (Fig.1). The protocol that we have used makes it possible to detect very weak cross-hybridizing signals. It is also clear from Figure 1 that there is essentially no detectable background in these experiments after 2 days of exposure. Prolonged exposure (up to 7 days) was used in subsequent experiments to ensure that no faintly hybridizing clones were missed. In these conditions non-specific background is detected.

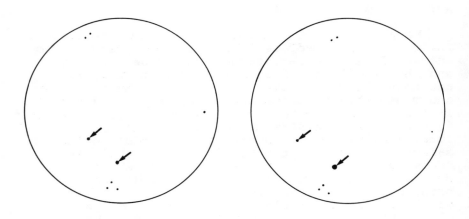

Figure 1 Primary screening of a chicken genomic library with a human HLA-DQ beta probe. Autoradiogram (2 day exposure) of duplicate filters showing two positive clones (arrows). The filters were marked with ink dots for positioning.

The identity of these clones has been verified by Northern and Southern blot analysis. DNA sequencing of one clone has shown that the hybridization with the HLA-DQ beta probe is due to a region containing exons for the beta 2 and transmembrane domains of a typical MHC class II beta chain gene (5). The hybridization conditions used allow detection of sequences sharing as low as 61% of their nucleotides with the probe. No false positives were obtained. This demonstrates the feasibility of the cross-hybridization approach and provides a point of entry to the chicken B complex.

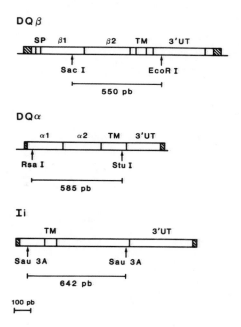

Figure 2 MHC class II probes. DQ beta: clone pDR beta 1 (8); DQ alpha: clone pDCH1 (9); Invariant chain: clone pGamma2 (10).

Attempts to isolate other MHC genes, the beta-2 microglobulin gene and the class II-associated invariant chain (Ii) gene.

Encouraged by the initial success in isolating the class II beta chain genes, we used a similar strategy to try to fish out the class II alpha chain gene and the class II-associated invariant chain gene. We were not able to obtain any positive clones in several independent experiments using a class II alpha chain probe and an invariant chain probe (Fig.2). In the case of the class II alpha chain, this might be related to the lower degree of conservation of class II alpha chains in mammals. It remains to be shown whether other human or murine class II alpha chain probes could be used successfully. The case of the invariant chain is more surprising since we have shown in biochemical studies of chicken B-L antigens that it is structurally well conserved (6).

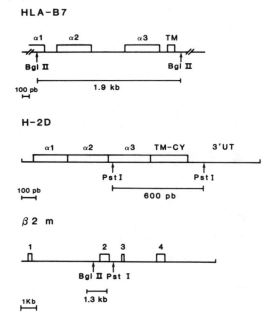

Figure 3 MHC class I probes. HLA-B7 gene (P.A. Birg and J. Strominger, unpublished); H-2 D : clone pH-2^d-33 (11); beta-2 microglobulin gene (H. Ploegh and J. Strominger, unpublished).

The failure to detect cross-hybridizing sequences with a murine beta-2 microglobulin probe (Fig.3) also indicates that the degree of sequence conservation observed between homologous sequences in mammals is not a precise indicator of the feasibility of the cross-hybridization approach.

The class I probes (Fig.3) that we have used contained the sequences coding for the last domains of the polypeptide chain. At best we were able to detect very faint bands by Southern blot analysis, but again failed to obtain positive clones by screening cDNA and genomic libraries.

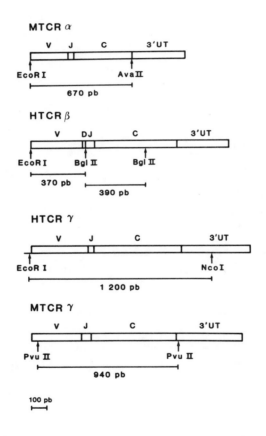

Figure 4 T-cell receptor probes. Mouse TCR alpha : clone Tl.2 (12); human TCR beta : clone HT beta (13); human TCR gamma : clone pTgammal (14); mouse TCR gamma : clone Tgamma5 (M. Steinmetz, unpublished).

Attempts to isolate T cell receptor and T cell differentiation antigen genes.

We have used a variety of cDNA probes corresponding to the T cell receptor alpha, beta and gamma chains (Fig.4), including variable and/or constant domain sequences as well as probes for the T3 delta chain and Thy-1 (Fig.5). As in the case of the MHC probes, the fragments used were devoid of GC rich segments and we had excluded the AT rich 3' untranslated regions. In all cases there was no detectable signal by Northern blot analysis or cDNA library screening.

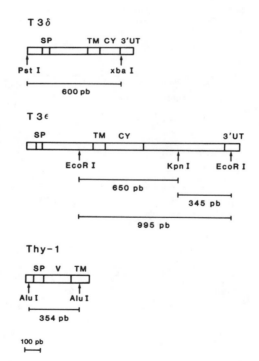

Figure 5 T-cell specific probes. T3 delta : clone pPGBC9 (15); T3 epsilon : clone pDJl (16); Thy-1 : clone pT64 (17).

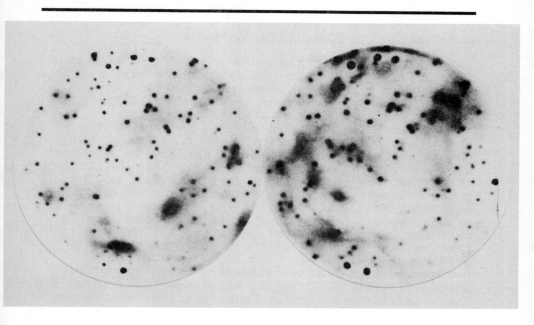

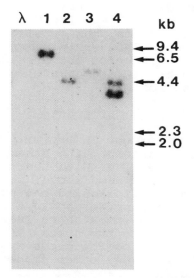

Figure 6 A phage clone (C4.3) hybridizing with a T3
epsilon probe. Top: duplicate filters of the final
screening. Bottom: Southern-blot analysis of the
phage clone. Lambda markers (no hybridization) Lane
1: C4.3 DNA cut with EcoRI, lane 2: Sac I, lane 3:
Ava I + EcoRI, lane 4: Sac I + Ava I.

The case of the T3 epsilon chain

The T3 epsilon chain probe (Fig.5) had been shown
to hybridize to chicken DNA by Southern blot analysis
(Cox Terhorst, personal communication) and we
directly used it to screen a genomic DNA library.
Several positive clones were isolated which
hybridized relatively strongly to the probe (Fig.6)
and to two adjacent subfragments from the probe. One
positive clone was purified and analyzed by Southern
blot and restriction enzyme analysis (Fig.3). It is
clear that the phage clone hybridizes well to the
probe. However we could not demonstrate any specific
messenger RNA hybridizing to the chicken sequence in
thymus, spleen or T cells. It is also worth noting
that the T3 epsilon probe was, among all the probes
that we have used, the most difficult to handle,
producing a relatively high background. This is
noticeable in the final screening of the purified
phages (Fig.6). In order to elucidate the nature of
the hybridizing sequence, we have tried to transfer
it into plasmid and M13 vectors. All our attempts were
unsuccessful, indicating that this sequence is highly
unstable in these vectors. At this stage we have
therefore no evidence that the isolated clone
contains the chicken T3 epsilon chain gene. Rather
these results reinforce our conviction that signals
detected by genomic Southern blot analysis cannot be
used as the sole criterion for predicting whether a
given probe can be used successfully in the cross-
hybridization approach.

Conclusions and future prospects

Except for the class II beta chain probe that we
used in our first attempt, the other probes have
yielded negative results. With the exception of the
T3 epsilon chain discussed above, we never obtained
false positives when following the protocol described
in the Methods section. We conclude at this stage
that the chicken sequences share less than 60% of
their nucleotides with the probes that we used. If
further attempts to use the cross-hybridization
approach are to be made, other probes and protocols
have to be used. For example a collection of T-cell
receptor V region probes could be used in the hope to
find one conserved subgroup similar to the
immunoglobulin VH III subgroup. However, when using a
rabbit V beta probe which is highly conserved in
mammals (7), we and others (Max Cooper, personal
communication) still failed to detect hybridization
signals. It might be possible to detect sequences

having less than 60% of their nucleotides in common with the probe by using RNA probes synthesized in vitro with SP6, T3 or T7 RNA polymerases.

In this report, we have summarized our experience accumulated over the past three years in attempting to obtain by the shortest route the chicken homologs of various MHC and T cell differentiation antigen genes. The cross-hybridization approach has provided a point of entry to the B complex and we have started to use the chromosome walking techniques to establish a molecular map of the chicken MHC. Antibodies recognizing the other gene products and biochemical information will probably serve as the basis for isolating the other genes.

Acknowledgments

We thank Patrice Marche, Per Peterson, Jack Silver, Michael Steinmetz, Jack Strominger, Cox Terhorst and their collaborators for providing the probes used in this study and Cox Terhorst and Max Cooper for sharing unpublished results. This work was supported by grants from Centre National de la Recherche Scientifique, Institut National de la Santé et de la Recherche Médicale and Association de la Recherche contre le Cancer to CA.

References

1 - Hood, L., Steinmetz, M. and Malissen, B. 1983. Genes of the major histocompatibility complex of the mouse. Ann. Rev. Immunol. 1 : 529-68.

2 - Auffray, C. and Strominger, J.L. 1986. Molecular genetics of the human major histocompatibility complex. Adv. Human Genet. 15 : 197-247.

3 - Longenecker, B.M. and Mosmann, T.R. 1981. Structure and properties of the major histocompatibility complex of the chicken. Speculations on the advantages and evolution of polymorphism. Immunogenetics 13 : 1-23.

4 - Davis, M.M., Chien, Y.H., Gascoigne, N.R.J. and Hedrick, S.M. 1984. A murine T cell receptor gene complex : isolation, structure and rearrangement. Immunol. Reviews 81 : 235-58.

5 - Bourlet, Y., Béhar, G., Guillemot, F. and Auffray, C. 1987. Isolation of a chicken major histocompatibility complex B-L beta gene : structure and expression in lymphoïd organs. Manuscript in preparation.

6 - Guillemot, F., Turmel, P., Charron, D., Le Douarin, N. and Auffray, C. 1986. Structure, biosynthesis and polymorphism of chicken MHC class II (B-L) antigens and associated molecules. J. Immunol. 137 : 1251-57.

7 - Marche, P. and Kindt, T. 1986. A variable region gene subfamily encoding T cell receptor beta chains is selectively conserved among mammals. J. Immunol. 137 : 1729-34.

8 - Larhammar, D., Schening, L., Gustaffson, K., Wiman, K., Claesson, L., Rask, L. and Peterson, P.A. 1982. Complete amino acid sequence of an HLA-DR antigen-like beta chain as predicted from the nucleotide sequence : similarities with immunoglobulins and HLA-A, -B and -C antigens. Proc. Natl. Acad. Sci. USA 79 : 3687-91.

9 - Auffray, C., Korman, A.J., Roux-Dosseto, M., Bono, R. and Strominger, J.L. 1982. cDNA clone for the heavy chain of the human B cell alloantigen DC1 : strong sequence homology to the HLA-DR heavy chain. Proc. Natl. Acad. Sci. 79 : 6337-41.

10 - Claeson, L., Larhammar, D., Rask, L. and
Peterson, P.A. 1983. cDNA clone for the human
invariant gamma chain of class II histocompatibility
antigens and its implications for the protein
structure. Proc. Natl. Acad. Sci. USA 80 : 7395-99.

11 - Lalanne, J.L., Delarbre, C., Gachelin, G. and
Kourilsky, P. 1983. cDNA containing the entire coding
sequence of a mouse H-2K^d histocompatibility antigen.
Nucleic Acids Res. 11 : 1567-77.

12 - Dembic, Z., Bannwarth, W., Taylor, B.A. and
Steinmetz, M. 1985. The gene encoding the T cell
receptor alpha chain maps to the Np-2 locus on mouse
chromosome 14. Nature 314 : 271-73.

13 - Jones, N., Leiden, J., Dialynas, D., Fraser, J.,
Clabby, M., Kishimoto, T. and Strominger, J.L. 1984.
Partial primary structure of the alpha and beta
chains of human tumors T cell receptor. Science 227 :
311-14.

14 - Quertermous, T., Murre, C., Dialynas, D., Duby,
A.D., Strominger, J.L., Waldman, T.A. and Seidman,
J.G. 1986. Human T-cell gamma chain genes :
organization, diversity and rearrangement. Science
231 : 252-55.

15 - van den Elsen, P., Stepley, B.A., Borst, J.,
Coligan, J.E., Markham, A.F., Orkin, S. and Terhorst,
C. 1984. Isolation of cDNA clones encoding the 20K T3
glycoprotein of human T-cell receptor complex. Nature
312 : 413-18.

16 - Gold, D.P., Puck, J.M., Pettey, C.L., Cho, M.,
Coligan, J., Woody, J.N. and Terhorst, C. 1986.
Isolation of cDNA clones encoding the 20K non-
glycosylated polypeptide chain of the human T-cell
receptor/T3 complex. Nature 321 : 431-34.

17 - Moriuchi, T., Chang, H.C., Denowe, R. and
Silver, J. 1983. Thy-1 cDNA sequence suggests a novel
regulatory mechanism. Nature 301 : 80-82.

RFLP Marker Genes for Physiologically and Serologically Identified Traits of the Equine MHC

Ernest Bailey, Jerold G. Woodward, Darrilyn G. Albright, and Alexander J. Alexander

DNA probes from human and mouse class I and class II genes cross-hybridized readily with restriction enzyme digested equine DNA to produce restriction fragment length polymorphisms (RFLP). Comparison of the RFLP markers to serological markers for the equine lymphocyte antigen (ELA) system demonstrated that the two methods identify genes in the same system. RFLP markers revealed more polymorphism than serology and distinguished different haplotypes for horses which are homozygous for serologically identified alleles. Susceptibility to sarcoid tumors and segregation distortion are two physiological traits associated with serological markers of the ELA system. Southern blot analysis was used to investigate RFLPs which might be more strongly associated with the traits. The murine class II probe pAAC6 for A alpha gene was hybridized with a blot of PVU II digested DNA from 10 horses which had sarcoid tumors. No evidence was found for a class II haplotype common to all horses. The murine pB1.4 probe for the murine TCP-1B gene was hybridized to PVU II digested DNA from 14 horses with different ELA types. All horses shared a common restriction fragment. A single variant band occurred for the only horse in the group which had the haplotype with the segregation distortion gene.

Introduction

The main premise for research on the major histocompatibility complex (MHC) of domestic animals is that fundamental immunologic mechanisms are controlled by MHC genes and that health related traits are often linked to the MHC. Lymphocyte alloantigens served as markers for the initial studies relating MHC and disease genes [1]. Recent studies demonstrated that DNA restriction fragment length polymorphisms (RFLP) analysis is well suited for the study of equine MHC markers and is also effective in studying disease associations with MHC genes [2,3].

We are interested in investigating the genetics of the equine MHC, particularly as it relates to health and physiology. Two physiological traits have been found associated with the equine MHC. First, sarcoid tumors are associated with the presence of the ELA-W13 specificity in several populations of horses [4-6]. Second, one haplotype of Standardbred horses exhibits segregation distortion from stallions, suggesting a

Bailey, Woodward, and Albright: Dept. of Vet. Sci., Maxwell H. Gluck Equine Res. Ctr., Univ. of Ky., Lexington, Ky. Woodward and Alexander: Dept. of Microbiol. and Immunol., Univ. of Ky., Lexington, Ky.

genetic influence on spermatogenesis or fertilization
[7].

The technique of Southern blot hybridization
reveals extensive polymorphism of the ELA system
beyond that detectable with lymphocyte typing. Human
and mouse probes for MHC genes were used to identify
class I, class II and class III genes of the horse [2,
8-10]. This technique promises to be an effective
tool for characterizing the genetics of the ELA
system, investigating MHC-associated health traits and
to guide us in improving ELA serology of class I and
class II genes.

Current status of equine MHC serology and genetics

In advance of Southern blot analysis of the equine
MHC, the ELA system had been identified serologically.
The ELA system encodes genes for lymphocyte alloantigens linked to the A blood group locus (1.6cM) and
with genes controlling responsiveness in mixed-
lymphocyte culture [11-14].

Four international workshops on the ELA system
have been held since 1981, involving participation
from 15 laboratories [15,16]. In the course of these
workshops 21 specificities were identified as products
of the ELA system. Eleven of those specificities
(A1-A10, W11) were clearly allelic products of a
single locus, designated ELA-A, and their distribution
has been studied in diverse horse breeds [16].

At least one additional ELA locus for alloantigens
has been identified based on recombinant haplotypes
discovered in two families. Lazary and co-workers
observed a recombinant haplotype among the offspring
of a stallion which showed that ELA-W13 was not a
product of the ELA-A locus [17]. Some data suggested
that ELA-W13 might even be a class II gene product.

Bernoco and co-workers observed a recombinant
haplotype among the offspring of another stallion in
which the loss of one specificity on the ELA haplotype
corresponded with appearance of another specificity
usually transmitted with the stallion's other haplotype [18]. They concluded that both specificities
were products of a putative ELA-B locus.

Bernoco and co-workers also observed another
recombinant within that family which allowed them to
map three loci of the ELA system in the order: A blood
group/ ELA-A/ ELA-B [18].

An important aspect of MHC research in the horse
is linkage disequilibrium for the ELA region. The A
blood group locus is 1.6 cM from the ELA-A locus and
yet strong linkage disequilibrium occurs for certain A

blood group alleles with certain ELA-A alleles [20].
     The expected frequencies for two non-allelic genes
occurring together is simply the product of their
phenotypic frequencies. When linkage disequilibrium
occurs, the observed frequencies will be much greater.
Table 1 lists the observed and expected haplotype
frequencies for three pairs of ELA-A:A blood group
alleles in Standardbred horses. ELA-A1 is strongly
associated with blood group Aa while ELA-W5 and
ELA-W10 are strongly associated with blood group Ab.
Strong linkage disequilibrium has also been reported
in another study of an ELA linked locus, namely equine
soluble class I substance.

TABLE 1. LINKAGE DISEQUILIBRIUM WITHIN THE EQUINE MHC.

Alleles in Linkage disequilibrium	Observed frequency	Expected frequency	reference
Standardbred			
ELA-A1, Aa	0.290	0.136	[20]
ELA-A5, Ab	0.139	0.074	[20]
ELA-A10, Ab	0.181	0.118	[20]
ELA-A4, ESCI+	0.120	0.036	[22]
ELA-A7, ESCI+	0.036	0.008	[22]
Thoroughbred			
ELA-A2, ESCI+	0.202	0.056	[22]

     Lew and co-workers identified a soluble class I
substance in horse serum (ESCI), analogous to the Q10
gene product in mice [21,22]. Soluble class I molecules were found in horses and related species but not
for dogs, cats, rats, hamsters, guinea pigs, ele-
phants, camels, elands, manatees, cattle, sheep, pigs
or goats. ESCI exhibited stronger linkage disequilibrium with ELA-A4 and A7 in Standardbred horses and
ELA-A2 in Thoroughbred horses than seen for the ELA-A
locus and the A blood group locus (Table 1).
     Linkage disequilibrium can be advantageous in
association studies. If we cannot identify the exact
gene responsible for a trait, a closely linked gene
can serve as a marker. Linked genes will segregate
with the trait in families and, when linkage disequilibrium exists, they will be associated with the
trait at the population level. The strength of the
association found between a marker and the trait will

depend on how closely linked the two genes are and the amount of linkage disequilibrium.

So far, serology of class II genes in the horse is not well developed. Aside from the problems of linkage disequilibrium, the distribution of class II genes in the horse may make it difficult to distinguish class I serology from class II serology. Class II antigens may be expressed on T lymphocytes in the horse. Monoclonal antibodies to class II epitopes recognize antigens on equine T lymphocytes as well as B lymphocytes [23]. As a consequence, it will be difficult to distinguish between class I and class II gene products using serology alone.

Fortunately, Southern blot hybridization appears to be a powerful method for studying the genetics of the equine MHC. DNA probes from human and mouse class I, class II and class III MHC genes cross-hybridize with horse DNA revealing many RFLPs [2, 8-10]. These markers offer a method for effective identification of diverse haplotypes which may be physiologically important.

RFLP analysis for class I genes

Vaiman and co-workers published the first Southern blots on the ELA system [8]. Class I genes were detected using a cross-hybridizing cDNA probe for the HLA-B7 gene and EcoRI digested DNA. They detected from 16 to 20 restriction fragments among each of five randomly selected horses with different serologically identified ELA types.

The first family studies using Southern blots of class I equine MHC genes were reported by Guerin and co-workers [9,10]. They also used a human probe for the HLA-B7 gene and restriction enzymes EcoRI, Hind III and Taq I. They observed 16 to 30 restriction fragments per horse with 3 polymorphic bands for EcoRI, 4 polymorphic bands for Hind III and 10 polymorphic bands for Taq I. Cosegregation of ELA alloantigens and class I RFLPs were observed in 18 instances in the two family studies reported by Guerin and co-workers, demonstrating that these tests are detecting markers for the ELA system

We have been particularly interested in characterizing class I genes of the horse and investigated modification of existing techniques to improve their identification. The methods are described elsewhere [2]. One problem with Southern blot analysis of ELA class I genes is the multiplicity of class I restriction fragments produced. To address this problem we used high resolution gel electrophoresis followed by

Southern blotting to increase separation between large DNA fragments. In an earlier study we selected 14 ELA-A locus homozygous Standardbred horses to further increase the expected differences between horses. RFLP patterns were highly correlated for those horses with the same ELA serotype, providing the first direct evidence that the ELA system is the equine MHC.

Using a murine class I cDNA probe and Hind III digestion of DNA we found 24 to 33 restriction fragments per horse, 14 of which were common to all horses. Pvu II enzyme digest yielded 23-30 restriction fragments per horse with 13 common bands. Similar results were produced when EcoRI was used as the restriction enzyme. In all three blots, most of the restriction fragments occurred in the region of the gel above 4.6 KB. Despite conditions to improve separation of the larger bands, separation still appeared incomplete.

No two horses were identical for all class I RFLPs despite homozygosity for ELA alloantigens. However, those with the same ELA type were more similar than those with different ELA types. Unique RFLPs for ELA-A1 and ELA-A6 were found in the Hind III blot.

Figure 1 shows a Southern blot using DNA from two sire families digested with Hind III restriction enzyme and hybridized with the murine class I probe after high resolution gel electrophoresis and blotting. More than 20 restriction fragments are present for all horses in this blot. However, only a few of those fragments exhibit polymorphism and show segregation in the families tested for this blot.

As described in the legend for Figure 1, the samples in this blot come from two sire-families. One stallion (P) is a standardbred stallion which was heterozygous for ELA-A5 and ELA-A8. His offspring which inherited the gene for ELA-A5 (haplotype a) also inherited the genes for RFLPs of approximately 6.3, 4.5 and 4.3 KB. No RFLPs were found associated with the ELA-A8 allele in this blot.

The second family included offspring of a Thoroughbred stallion (p). He was homozygous for the ELA-A2 alloantigen. However, as can be seen in Figure 1, he appeared to be heterozygous for ELA markers detected as RFLPs. His offspring inherited the genes for RFLPs of 10.2, 5.7, 4.5 and 4.3 KB or the gene for a single RFLP of approximately 3.6 KB.

In this case the haplotype differences detected by Southern blotting in this Thoroughbred family reflected alloantigenic variation which previously had been undetected. Recently we produced antisera to a specificity unique to one of these two ELA-A2

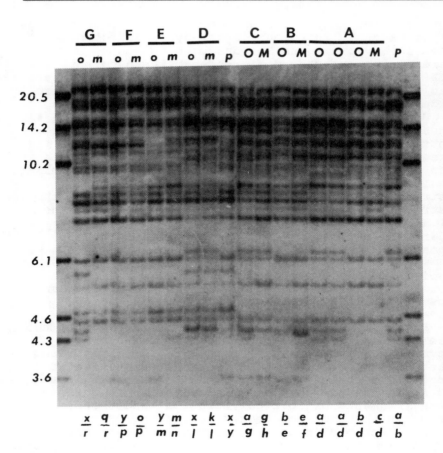

FIGURE 1. Autoradiogram of Southern blot for equine
DNA digested with Hind III restriction enzyme and
probed with murine class I cDNA probe. The capital
letters (A-G) at the top of the figure identify sets
of dams and offspring. Below those letters the dams
are identified with "M" or "m"; offspring are identified with "O" or "o". The lane representing the sire
of all offspring denoted with "O" is denoted "P" at
the top of the left-most lane in the figure. The lane
for the sire of offspring denoted with "o" is denoted
"p" at the top of one of the middle lanes in the
figure. The ELA haplotypes of the parental horses are
represented with letters a-x at the bottom of the
figure as follows: a/b = A5/A8; c/d = A4/A10; e/f =
A4/A10; g/h = A4/A10; x/y=A2#/A2*; k/l=A2/A3;
m/n=A1/A3; o/p=A1/W11; q/r=A2/W11.

haplotypes by immunizing the stallion's offspring with white blood cells from the stallion (unpublished data).

While the number of RFLPs seen in Figure 1 is less than that described by Alexander and co-workers using the same methods, it is comparable to the results of Guerin and co-workers who also studied families of ELA-A heterozygous horses [2,9,10].

The complexity of the equine class I genes causes Southern blotting analysis to be cumbersome. It appears unlikely that RFLPs showing a one-to-one correspondence with ELA alloantigens will be found easily. On the other hand, our preliminary studies indicate that clusters of RFLPs correlate well with ELA haplotypes and are generally predictive of the ELA type. The focus of further studies on class I genes should be to increase separation of the large DNA fragments and to clone more specific probes for class I genes which recognize a more restricted subset of RFLPs.

RFLP analysis for equine class II genes

Class II serology, as such, does not exist for the horse. While 21 antigenic determinants have been recognized as products of ELA genes, it is not known in most cases whether they are products of class I or class II genes.

Human class II probes are effective in Southern blot hybridization of horse DNA. Vaiman and co-workers used human probes to DR beta and DQ alpha genes in their study of Eco RI digested DNA from five horses. They found 15 to 20 restriction fragments per horse using the DR beta probe and 5 to 7 bands using the DQ alpha probe [8].

Guerin and co-workers used probes for human genes DR beta and DQ alpha in Southern blot studies on Eco RI, Hind III and Taq I DNA digests for a family of horses [9,10]. The segregation of RFLPs coincided with the segregation of ELA serological markers. EcoRI and Taq I digests using the DR beta probe yielded 9 to 11 bands per individual with 5 polymorphic bands; Hind III digests showed 11 bands with 6 polymorphic bands. The DQ alpha probe detected 9, 10 and 13 restriction fragments respectively with EcoRI, Hind III and Taq I enzyme digestion; Of these bands, 7, 9 and all 13 were polymorphic, respectively.

Alexander and co-workers used mouse class II probes to study restriction enzyme digested DNA from 14 homozygotes for serologically identified ELA genes [2]. A single, non-polymorphic band was produced for

the E-alpha gene using Pvu II digestion. This is
consistent with other species in which the E alpha
gene is present as a single non-polymorphic gene. A
cDNA probe for A alpha was effective in identifying 3
to 5 strongly hybridizing bands per horse with none of
the bands common to all horses, ie, all bands were
polymorphic.

Two genomic probes for E-beta and A-beta were used
which contained the entire class II sequence. Multiple
polymorphic bands were found however, the similarity
between blots with these two probes suggested that
they did not adequately distinguish between the
equivalent loci for E beta and A beta of the horse.

The type of patterns found for the class II RFLPs
were similar overall to those seen for the class I
genes, ie, horses with the same ELA types were usually
more similar than those with different ELA types. This
is consistent with linkage of ELA class I with class
II genes and linkage disequilibrium.

The exceptions to this rule were the class II
RFLPs seen for the ELA-A1 and ELA-A10 homozygous
horses. Blots with Pvu II digested DNA were probed
with genomic DNA probes for A-beta and E-beta chains
and a cDNA probe for E-alpha chain. The two ELA-A1
and one of the two ELA-A10 horses had identical RFLP
patterns for each of the three radiographs. The other
ELA-A10 horse had no bands in common for one radio-
graph (E-alpha probe) but shared some bands on the
other two radiographs. Presumably the three horses
with the same RFLP pattern had a common class II gene
region.

Although different for class II RFLPs the two
horses with ELA-A10 were very similar for the class I
RFLP patterns. Therefore, the difference between the
two ELA-A10 horses may be due to a recombination of
the haplotype for one of their ancestors which separated the class I and class II regions of the ances-
tor's haplotype. As a consequence this difference
provides additional evidence that the serology of the
ELA-A locus is directed against class I gene products
and not class II gene products, at least as far as
ELA-A1 and ELA-A10 are concerned. It will be useful
in the future to combine the results of Southern blot
studies with functional studies such as mixed lymphocyte culture responses.

In summary, class II probes from humans and mice
cross-hybridize well with equine DNA. Southern blots
were effective in identifying polymorphism for the ELA
region class II genes and indicated that considerable
polymorphism exists. In all three studies, most of
the restriction fragments were polymorphic. However,

insufficient work has been done to consider the number
of class II genes or their homology to DR, DQ, DP, I-A
or I-E loci. Given the difficulty of serologically
testing for class II genes, molecular techniques
clearly offer a solution for studying class II genes
in the horse.

Sarcoid tumors and association with ELA markers

In the horse, sarcoid tumors are benign fibroblas-
tic dermal tumors which are thought to be caused by a
retrovirus [24]. Lazary and co-workers reported the
association of ELA-W13 with the presence of sarcoid
tumors in the horse [4]. This study was repeated and
confirmed for Thoroughbred horses [5]. ELA-W13 is
strongly associated with ELA-A3 at the population
level but can occur with other ELA-A locus alloantigens. Antisera to anti-W13 blocked responses of cells
in mixed-lymphocyte-culture suggesting that it might
also be a class II gene product [17].

The association of sarcoid tumors with ELA-W13 is
not complete, ie, some animals without the ELA-W13
specificity develop sarcoid tumors. One possibility
is that ELA-W13 is not the gene responsible for
susceptibility, but rather linked to another gene
which is actually responsible for sarcoid tumor
susceptibility. This is supported by the observation
that some families show segregation of different ELA
alleles with the occurrence of sarcoid tumors [6]. We
should be able to find another marker which is even
more closely associated with sarcoid tumor susceptibility. To investigate this possibility we did Southern blot analysis on DNA collected from horses with
sarcoid tumors to see if an RFLP marker might be more
strongly associated with the presence of sarcoid
tumors of the horse.

Local veterinarians generously provided us with
blood samples from 15 Thoroughbred horses known to
have had sarcoid tumors. While 32% of randomly
selected Thoroughbred horses possessed the ELA-A3,W13
haplotype, 9 of 15 (60%) of the sarcoid affected
horses possessed that haplotype. This is consistent
with results of the previous two reports on association of sarcoid tumors with ELA types [4,5].

DNA was isolated from 10 of these horses, digested
with Pvu II restriction enzyme and used for Southern
blot analysis. The blot was hybridized with the pAAc6
murine class II A-alpha chain probe. A class II probe
was chosen because of previous suggestion that ELA-W13
might be a class II gene product and this marker is
most strongly associated with the presence of sarcoid

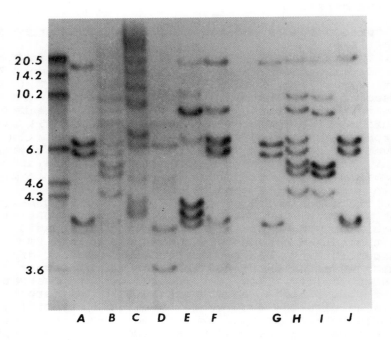

FIGURE 2. Autoradiogram of Southern blot for equine
DNA digested with Pvu II restriction enzyme and
hybridized with murine A-alpha chain probe pAAc6. All
horses represented in this blot had sarcoid tumors.
The ELA types of the horses for each lane were as
follows: A= A3,W13; B=A2; C=A3,W13; D=A3,W13/A6; E=
A5/W11; F=A3,W13/A9; G=A3,W13; H=A2/A9; I=A2;
J=A3,W13.

tumors.

As can be seen in Figure 2, there is not a single common pattern of RFLPs among these horses. While there is a common band at approximately 6.1 KB, this band is also common in other Pvu II digests probed with the pAAc6 probe [2, unpublished data]. The horses represented in lanes a, c, d, f, g and i possessed the W13 antigens on their lymphocytes and might be expected to have a common RFLP pattern. The horse in lane d clearly did not exhibit that pattern.

Several patterns were apparent and related to ELA types. One pattern in lanes a, c, f, g and i included RFLPs of approximately 6.2, 6.0, and 4.0 KB common to a subset of horses with ELA-A3,W13. Likewise, there is a pattern entirely unique to those horses with ELA-A2 in lanes b, h, and i (approximately 5.5, 5.3 and 4.3 KB). In any case, and under these conditions, it does not appear that any of the RFLPs are better markers for susceptibility to sarcoid tumors than serological detection of ELA-W13.

More information is needed before firm conclusions are drawn. Assuming a common origin of the suscepti-bility gene and assuming linkage disequilibrium of the class II gene region, most enzymes and most class II probes should produce a common pattern if the gene were within this region. On the other hand the gene for susceptibility to sarcoid tumors may be included within different large RFLPs and require a different restriction enzyme to reveal a common pattern.

RFLP markers for the MHC segregation distorter gene

While much attention on the MHC and MHC linked genes involves the search for immune response genes or disease susceptibility genes, there is another MHC linked gene complex of interest, namely the t-complex of the mouse. Studies on mouse and rat MHC genes demonstrated that the MHC of those species includes genes which influence reproduction and development [25-27]. Since the MHC linkage group appears to be roughly conserved throughout evolution, it is possible that all vertebrate species possess MHC genes which influence reproduction and development.

The murine t-complex is actually quite unique and it is unlikely that an identical complex exists in other species. All t-complex haplotypes found in the mouse are descendant from a chromosome containing two inversions within the MHC region. Depending upon the genotype, t-genes will cause segregation distortion in the male, embryonic loss, male sterility and even

skeletal defects affecting primarily the tail. Nevertheless, these unique haplotypes tell us that genes
influencing fertility and development are present
within or linked to the MHC.

Recently we found evidence for a trait in the
horse which is similar to one of the t-complex traits,
namely male segregation distortion [7]. A stallion
and 15 of his 17 sons transmitted the ELA-A10 haplotype to offspring more frequently than their allelic
haplotype. For all stallions possessing that haplotype, ELA-A10 was transmitted 368 times as compare to
270 times for allelic haplotypes (P=0.0001). While
this represents only a 57.7% transmission as compared
to greater than 90% transmission of most t-haplotypes
in the mouse, these data are highly significant and
reproducible between farms and between years.

In order to determine whether this trait is
analogous to the genes associated with the t-complex,
we obtained a cDNA probe for one of the products of
the t-complex. Dr. Keith Willison generously provided
the pB1.4 cDNA clone for one of the t-complex
products, TCP-1B [28].

This probe effectively cross-hybridized with
equine DNA. As can be seen in Figure 3, restriction
enzyme digest of DNA from two horses with different
ELA types using the enzymes Eco RI, Pvu II, Bam Hl and
Hind III and probed with pB1.4 revealed one or two
strong restriction fragments with additional faint
bands visible. No differences were seen between these
two horses. A blot with Pvu II digested DNA, previously reported by Alexander and co-workers, was
reprobed with pB1.4 and is shown in Figure 4. All
horses had a common restriction fragment at 5.5 KB. A
single variant band, approximately 4.0 KB, was
observed for DNA from one horse (*). This horse was
also the only horse possessing the ELA-A10 haplotype
associated with segregation distortion. Although the
evidence is circumstantial at this point, it strongly
suggests that we have found a gene marker useful to
identify haplotypes with the gene causing segregation
distortion. Family studies will provide a definite
answer.

CONCLUSION

In advance of Southern blot hybridization studies
in the horse only a single locus of the ELA system was
well characterized. Southern blot studies showed, for
the first time, that there were clearly a multiplicity
of loci for class I and class II genes in the horse.

Class I blots of the horse reveal complexity which

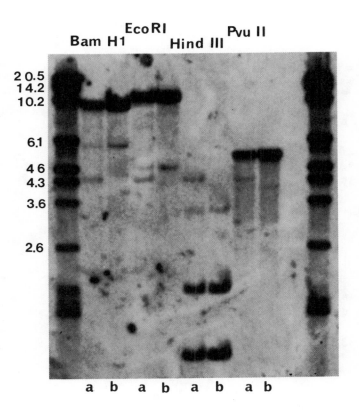

Figure 3. Autoradiogram of Southern blot of horse
leukocyte DNA hybridized with a 790 base pair cDNA
probe (pB1.4) to the murine gene Tcp-1. As indicated
above the lanes, restriction enzymes Bam H1, Eco RI,
Hind III and Pvu II were used. Lanes designated a
correspond to DNA from a Standardbred horse type
ELA-A4/A10; Lanes designated b correspond to DNA from
a Standardbred horse type ELA-A5/A8. Kilobase standards are derived from a Bam H1/Eco RI digestion of
Adenovirus-2 DNA.

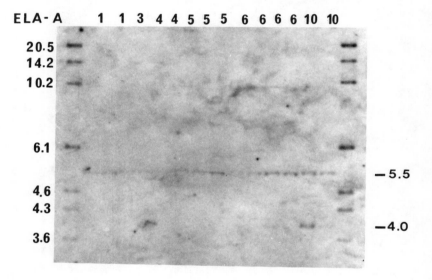

Figure 4. Pvu II Southern blot of horse leukocyte DNA hybridized with pB1.4. All horses were homozygous for ELA-A alloantigens. ELA type is indicated above each lane. An * appears below the lane of the single horse which possessed the RFLP of approximately 4.0 KB.

shall be difficult to unravel without a concerted and
methodical approach. Use of diverse restriction
enzymes, modifying the conditions of electrophoresis
and development and use of new gene probes can trans-
form a non-informative mating into an informative one
by revealing new RFLPs. The level of polymorphism
appears great.

Southern blotting identified polymorphism between
haplotypes which are serologically indistinguishable.
This will also be useful in parentage studies. Lymphocyte typing is already one of the most effective tests
for identifying incorrect parentage in horse [29].
This is based on the high level of heterozygosity for
the genes encoding alloantigens of the ELA system.
RFLPs clearly reveal even greater heterozygosity for
the ELA system.

Southern blots will clearly be useful in unravel-
ling the class II gene system in the horse. If class
II genes are expressed on T lymphocytes of the horse,
then it will be exceedingly difficult to make serological distinction between class I and class II gene
products. Serology will have to develop in coupling
with, or following, molecular characterizations of the
MHC class II genes of the horse.

It is now possible to directly identify ELA genes
that encode the serologically detectable molecules for
ELA genes for which we have antisera. By isolating
full length cDNA or genomic clones from horse lymphocyte libraries followed by transfection and expression
in mouse L cells, it will be possible to directly
equate a serological specificity with the gene that
encodes it.

Finally, Southern blot studies provide a powerful
method to verify association of physiological traits
with the MHC. As reviewed here, the ELA system is
certainly complex and linkage disequilibrium affects
its use in association studies. When the gene marker
is loosely linked to the gene in question, linkage
disequilibrium allows us to detect the association
within a breed and particularly within a family.
However, Southern blot analysis allows us to search
for RFLP markers which may show even stronger associations with the trait and even map the location of the
haplotype associated gene.

ACKNOWLEDGEMENTS: These studies have been funded by
The Jockey Club Research Foundation, The Grayson
Foundation, NIH grant R01 HD 14487 and in connection
with a project of The Kentucky Agricultural Experiment
Station (paper No. 87-4-247). The authors are grateful to Ms. Ann Marie Rossi for excellent technical
support.

REFERENCES

1. Svejgaard, A., P. Platz and L.P. Ryder. 1983. HLA
    and disease. A survey. Immunological Reviews 70:
    193-218.

2. Alexander, A.J., E. Bailey, J.G. Woodward. 1987.
    Analysis of the equine lymphocyte antigen system
    by Southern blot hybridization. Immunogenetics 25:
    47-54.

3. Marcadet, A., C. Massart, G. Semana, R. Fauchet,
    O. Sabraud, M. Merienne, J. Dausset and D. Cohen.
    1985. Association of class II HLA-DQ beta chain
    DNA restriction fragments with multiple sclerosis.
    Immunogenetics 22: 93-96.

4. Lazary, S., H. Gerber, P.A. Glatt and R. Straub.
    1985. Equine leukocyte antigens in sarcoid
    affected horses. Equine Veterinary Journal 17:
    283-286.

5. Meredith, D., A.H. Elser, B. Wolf, L.R. Soma, W.J.
    Donawick and S. Lazary. 1986. Equine leukocyte
    antigens: relationships with sarcoid tumors and
    laminitis in two pure breeds. Immunogenetics 23:
    221-225.

6. Gerber, H., M.-L. Dubath and S. Lazary. 1987.
    Association between predisposition to equine
    sarcoid and the MHC in multiple case families.
    Proceedings of the Fifth International Conference
    on Equine Infectious Diseases. Lexington, KY. in
    press.

7. Bailey, E. 1986. Segregation distortion within the
    equine MHC; analogy to a murine T/t complex trait.
    Immunogenetics 24: 225-229.

8. Vaiman, M., P. Chardon and D. Cohen. 1986. DNA
    polymorphism in the major histocompatibility
    complex of man and various farm animals. Animal
    Genetics 17: 113-134.

9. Guerin, G., M. Bertaud, P. Chardon, C. Geffrotin,
    M. Vaiman and D. Cohen. 1987. Molecular genetic
    analysis of the major histocompatibility complex
    in an ELA typed horse family. Animal Genetics (in
    press).

10. Guerin, G., H. Varewyck, M. Bertaud and P.
    Chasset. 1987. Analysis of a horse family with a
    crossing over between the ELA complex and the A
    blood group system. Animal Genetics (in press).

11. Bailey, E., C. Stormont, Y. Suzuki and A.
    Trommershausen-Bowling. 1979. Linkage of loci
    controlling alloantigens on red blood cells and
    lymphocytes in the horse. Science 204: 1317-1319.

12. Lazary, S., A.L. deWeck, S. Bullen, R. Straub and
    H. Gerber. 1980. Equine leukocyte antigen system.
    I. Serological studies. Transplantation 30:
    203-209.

14. Antczak, D.F., S.M. Bright, L.H. Remick and B.E.
    Bauman. 1982. Lymphocyte alloantigens of the
    horse. 1. Serologic and genetic studies. Tissue
    Antigen 20: 172-180.

13. Lazary, S. S. Bullen, J. Muller, G. Kovacs, I.
    Bodo, P. Hockenjos and A.L. deWeck. 1980. Equine
    leukocyte antigen system. II. Serological and
    mixed-lymphocyte reactivity studies in families.
    Transplantation 30: 210-215.

15. Bull, R.W. (ed). 1983. Joint report of the first
    international conference on lymphocyte
    alloantigens of the horse, held 24-29 October
    1981. Animal Blood Groups and Biochemical Genetics
    14: 119-137.

16. Bernoco, D., D.F. Antczak, E. Bailey, K. Bell,
    R.W. Bull, G. Byrns, G.Guerin, S.Lazary, J.
    McClure, J. Templeton and H. Varewyck. 1987. Joint
    report of the fourth international workshop on
    lymphocyte alloantigens of the horse, Lexington,
    Kentucky, 12-22 October 1985. Animal Blood Groups
    and Biochemical Genetics 18: 81-94.

17. Lazary, S., M.-L. Dubath, Ch. Luder and H. Gerber.
    1986. Equine leukocyte antigen system. IV.
    Recombination within the major histocompatibility
    complex (MHC). Journal of Immunogenetics 13:315-325.

18. Bernoco, D., G. Byrns, E. Bailey and A.M. Lew. 1987. Evidence of a second polymorphic ELA class I (ELA-B) locus and gene order for three loci of the equine MHC. Animal Genetics 18: 103-118.

19. Fries, R., R. Hediger, H.A. Ansari, D.J.S. Hetzel and G. Stranzinger. 1987. Chromosomal assignment of the major histocompatibility complex in swine, cattle and horse by in situ hybridization.(abstract) Ninth International Conference on Human Gene Mapping, Paris. (in press).

20. Bailey, E. 1983. Linkage disequilibrium between the ELA and A blood group systems in American Standardbred horses. Animal Blood Groups and Biochemical Genetics 14: 119-137.

21. Lew, A.M., R.B. Valas, W.L. Maloy and J.E. Coligan. 1986. A soluble class I molecule analogous to mouse Q10 in the horse and related species. Immunogenetics 23: 277-283.

22. Lew, A.M., E. Bailey, R.B. Valas and J.E. Coligan. 1986. The gene encoding the equine soluble class I molecule is linked to the horse MHC. Immunogenetics 24: 128-130.

13. Crepaldi, T., A. Crump, M. Newman, S. Ferrone and D.F. Antczak. 1986. Equine T lymphocytes express MHC class II antigens. Journal of Immunogenetics. 13: 349-360.

24. Cheevers, W.P., S.M. Robertson, A.L. Brassfield, W.C. Davis and T.B. Crawford. 1982. Isolation of a retrovirus from cultured equine sarcoid tumor cells. American Journal of Veterinary Research 43: 804-806.

25. Bennett, D. 1975. The T-locus of the mouse. Cell 6: 441-454.

26. Gill, T.J. and H.W. Kunz. 1979. Gene complex controlling growth and fertility linked to the major histocompatibility complex in the rat. American Journal of Pathology 96: 185-205.

27. Warner, C.M., S.O. Gollnick, L. Flaherty and S.B. Goldbard. 1987. Analysis of Qa-2 antigen

expression by preimplantation mouse embryos:
possible relationship to the
preimplantation-embryo-development (Ped) gene
product. Biology of Reproduction 36: 611-616.

28. Willison, K.R., K. Dudley and J. Potter. 1986.
Molecular cloning and sequence analysis of a
haploid expressed gene encoding t complex
polypeptide 1. Cell 44: 727-738.

29. Bailey, E. 1984. Usefulness of lymphocyte typing
to solve incorrectly assigned paternity in horses.
American Journal of Veterinary Research 45:
1979-1983.

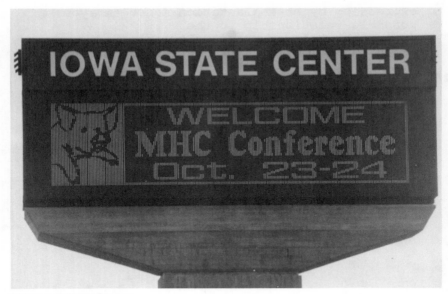
Welcome to the conference

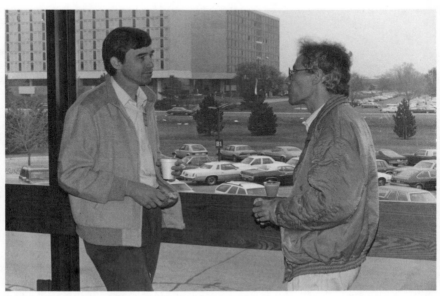
Ernie Bailey and Gerard Guerin discuss the day's events

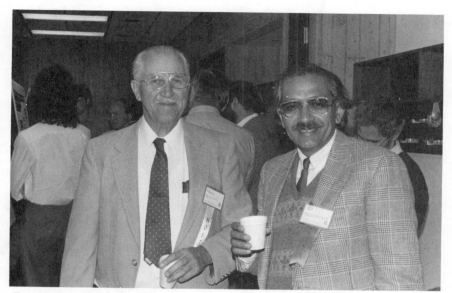

"Two roosters" view poster session

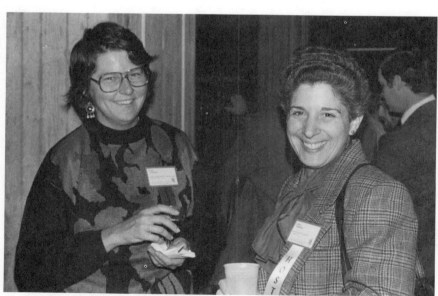

Joan Lunney and Carol Warner at the reception

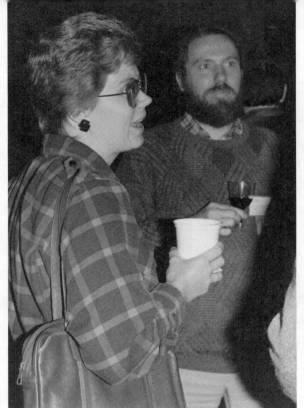

**Susan Lamont
and Charles Auffray**

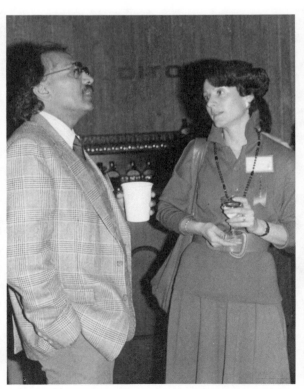

**Dinah Singer
and Chella David**

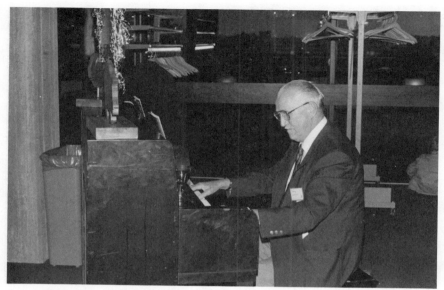

Arne Nordskog entertains his colleagues

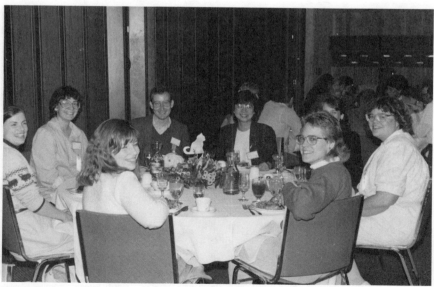

ISU hosts take a rest

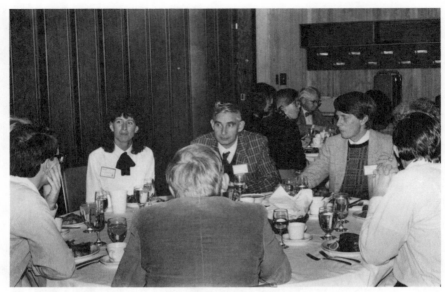

Noel Muggli, Marcel Vaiman, Patrick Chardon, and others enjoy the banquet

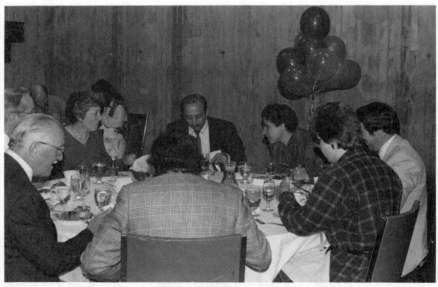

Richard and Esther Willham, Max Rothschild, Carol Warner, Steve Ford, Susan Lamont, Chella David, and Arne Nordskog

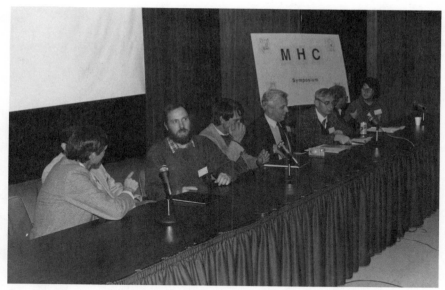

Arne Nordskog receives his award for Distinguished MHC Research at Iowa State University

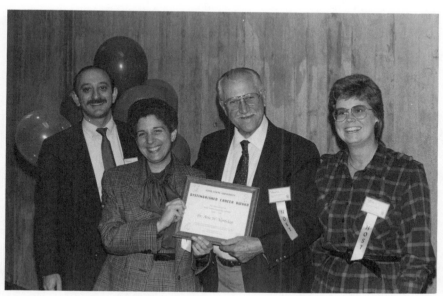

Panel discussion with symposium speakers

PART 2

Abstracts

1   Serological and biochemical analysis of the major histocompati-
    lity complex of the chicken (B-complex).
JAN J BLANKERT*, RIA VRIELINK, IRMA ENGELEN, MARCEL GJ
TILANUS*.   Agricultural University, Wageningen, the Netherlands.

In the present study we characterized the polymorphism of separate
loci of the B-complex in two lines of White Leghorn chickens (31 and 7
individuals respectively). Direct hemagglutination was performed using
class I (B-F) and class IV (B-G) specific alloantisera. DNA-polymorphism
of class II (B-L) genes was determined in Southern blot analysis using
cross-hybridizing human cDNA subprobes. Serological typing revealed
the presence of B19, B21 and B34 haplotypes in both lines. These
haplotypes contained co-segregating B-F and B-G allotypes. In Southern
blot analysis four different class II fragments were identified with the
cDNA probes. However, the restriction fragment length polymorphism
(RFLP) did not correlate with the serological class I/IV typing results.
Apparently, individuals which have serologically identical B-F and B-G
products, may have different class II genes. Further studies will be
performed to analyze polymorphism of class II as well as class I genes
in relation with the serological characterization of class I and class II
products.

2   Restriction Fragment Length Polymorphism (RFLP) Analysis
    of Chicken MHC Class II (B-L) Genes of Fourteen Iowa State
University Inbred Lines   BRADLEY M. GERNDT*[1], SUSAN J. LAMONT[2],
YUANXIN XU[1], CHARLES AUFFRAY[3], YVES BOURLET[3], A.W. NORDSKOG[2],
CAROL M. WARNER[1] [1]Departments of Biochemistry-Biophysics and
[2]Animal Science, Iowa State University, Ames, Iowa 50011 USA
[3]Institut d'Embryologie' du CNRS et du College de France, Nogent
S/Marne, France

RFLP analysis was conducted on sperm DNA of 4 chickens from
each of 14 highly-inbred, serologically defined MHC haplotypes.
White Leghorn, Egyptian, and Spanish breeds, and MHC haplotypes
1, 5.1, 6, 12, 13, 15, 15.1, and 15.2 were represented. Two
chicken MHC Class II β probes were used. Restriction enzymes
Pvu II and Bam HI yielded extensive polymorphisms, whereas Eco
RI and Hind III digests were less informative. RFLP patterns of
individuals of the same B blood type within a line were identical. Some patterns, however, differed between individuals of
the same B blood type in different lines, and also between different B blood types within lines. This study demonstrates that
analysis of Class II genes can give additional information about
MHC types of chickens, beyond that obtained with serological B
blood group typing.

3   Restriction Fragment Length Polymorphism (RFLP) Analysis
      of the Major Histocompatibility Class II ß Genes of
15I₅-B Congenic Chicken Lines. SUSAN J. LAMONT,[*1] BRADLEY M.
GERNDT,[2] CAROL M. WARNER[2], and LARRY D. BACON[3]. [1]Department of
Animal Science, and [2]Department of Biochemistry and Biophysics,
Iowa State University, Ames, IA 50011. [3]USDA-ARS-Regional
Poultry Research Laboratory, 3606 Mount Hope Road, East
Lansing, MI 48823.

       Samples of DNA from whole blood of three birds from each
of five 15I₅-B-homozygous congenic lines were analysed by RFLP.
The probe used was a chicken MHC class II ß clone (kindly
provided by Dr. C. Auffray, CNRS, France). Digestion of DNA
with Hind III yielded three nonpolymorphic bands. Pvu II
digestion yielded two different patterns of four bands each,
with one polymorphic band. One individual's DNA exhibited two
polymorphic bands, suggesting heterozygosity of Class II ß
genes. This individual's heterozygosity was subsequently
confirmed by blood typing. BamHI digestion yielded two
patterns of four bands each, with one polymorphic band. One
bird's DNA showed two polymorphic bands, and another showed no
polymorphic bands, suggesting some variation in the MHC Class
II ß genes not detectable upon serological B typing.

4   Analysis of the S1 Chicken Line by Hybridization of
       Sperm DNA to an MHC Class II Probe. Jacob Pitcovski[*1],
Susan J. Lamont[2], Arne W. Nordskog[2], Bradley M. Gerndt[1], Carol
M. Warner[1]. [1]Dept. of Biochemistry/Biophysics and [2]Dept. of
Animal Science, Iowa State University, Ames, Iowa 50011 USA.

       Sperm DNA was isolated from S1 chickens which were sero-
logically typed to be B^1B^1, $B^{19}B^{19}$ or B^1B^{19}. The DNA was
digested with a number of different restriction enzymes and
subjected to Southern blot analysis with a probe directed to a
class II gene of the major histocompatability complex (kindly
provided by Dr. Charles Auffray, CNRS, France). Restriction
fragment length polimorphisms (RFLPs) were found in the DNA
isolated from B^1B^1 and $B^{19}B^{19}$ chickens when the DNA was cut by
Sau3A, BglII, PvuII and TaqI. No differences were found
between the lines when EcoRI was used as a restriction enzyme.
Analysis of heterozygous chickens, B^1B^{19}, showed that all bands
were inherited in a Mendalian fashion. This study shows that
RFLP analysis of chicken DNA may be a useful alternative to
serological testing for MHC haplotype.

5   Restriction Fragment Length Polymorphisms in the Bovine Major
Histocompatibility Class II Genes using Homologous Probes. MUGGLI,
NOELLE E.* and ROGER T. STONE, USDA-ARS, RLH U.S. Meat Animal Research Center,
P.O. Box 166, Clay Center, Nebraska 68933.

Bovine DNA was digested with EcoRI and hybridized with homologous probes
after Southern transfer. The first probe, 8-2 β2/TM, was a 1.0 kb PstI/BamHI
fragment from a bovine genomic clone that crosshybridized to cDNA HLA DRβ. The
fragment was sequenced and contained a DRβ-like β2 exon, an .8 kb intron and a
DRβ-like transmembrane (TM) exon. Hybridization with this probe results in 7
bands; 18.9, 7.2, 6.4, 5.6, 3.6, 3.0 and 2.7 kb. All but the 18.9 kb band were
polymorphic. The 3.6 kb band corresponds to the β2 and TM-containing EcoRI
fragment from the genomic clone. Loss of the 5' EcoRI site from the 3.6 kb
fragment would result in the 5.6 kb band. The second probe, 9 TM, was a 1.3 kb
PstI fragment from another bovine genomic clone and contained a DRβ-like TM
exon. Hybridization with this probe resulted in two codominant bands, 6.4 and
3.7 kb. The occurrence of these two bands for each animal tested was the same
as the occurrence of the 6.4 and 2.7 kb bands using the 8-2 β2/TM probe. Under
these hybridization conditions, the 8-2 β2/TM probe apparently crosshybridizes
to the 9 β2 exon while the TM exons do not. We suggest there is a polymorphic
EcoRI site within the 6.4 kb fragment and between the 9 β2 and TM exons. When
the site is present, two fragments are created; a 2.7 kb fragment containing
the β2 exon and a 3.7 kb fragment containing the TM exon. Thus, EcoRI RFLPs
have been identified for two bovine Class II DRβ-like genes.

6   Polymorphism Among Serologically-Defined BoLA Class I
Homozygotes Revealed by RFLP Analysis JULIE A. STEWART*,
LAWRENCE B. SCHOOK, and HARRIS A. LEWIN. Department of Animal
Sciences, University of Illinois, Urbana, Il. 61801.

Although polymorphic BoLA class I antigens are readily
detected serologically, reagents for detecting polymorphic class
II antigens are more difficult to produce. Since class II
molecules are important in immune responsiveness, we were
interested in studying polymorphism of class II genes in BoLA
haplotypes bearing w20, a common class I allele in the Holstein-
Friesian breed (gene freq. 16.6%). To determine if BoLA-A locus
(class I) alleles are associated with different class II
alleles, four Holstein-Friesian BoLA w20 homozygotes were
tested for polymorphism in the DQα gene by Southern blot
analysis using a 560bp RsaI/StuI fragment of a human cDNA probe,
pDCHI. Genomic DNA from three w20 homozygous paternal half-sibs
and one unrelated w20 homozygote was digested with the
restriction enzyme PvuII and hybridized with the DQα probe. Six
common fragments were seen in each sample. One of the half-
sibs, however, exhibited a 2.5Kb RFLP not present in the other
w20 homozygotes, thus demonstrating variation in BoLA
haplotypes. (Supported by USDA Proposal # 8701469)

7   Genetic variability between two breeds based on
      restriction endonuclease fragment polymorphisms of
major histocompatibility complex class I genes in swine.
YOUNG C. JUNG*, MIKE FLANAGAN, MAX F. ROTHSCHILD, CAROL M.
WARNER. Dept. of Animal Science and Dept. of Biochemistry
and Biophysics. Iowa State University, Ames, Iowa, USA.

Restriction fragment length polymorphism (RFLP) analyses
of SLA class I genes were performed on 70 Duroc and 38
Hampshire boars from the 1986-7 national performance tests.
Few boars were inbred. Southern blotting and hybridization
procedures were performed using PvuII endonuclease and the
PD1-A swine MHC class I probe (kindly provided by Dr. Dinah
Singer, NIH). The Duroc breed produced an average of 11
restriction fragments averaging 5.0 kb (1.3-12.5 kb). The
Hampshire breed produced an average of 12 restriction
fragments averaging 3.3 kb (1.1-14.3 kb). Nucleotide
diversity, which represents the average number of nucleotide
differences per site between two DNA sequences, was
calculated. The nucleotide diversities of Durocs, Hampshires
and between breeds were 0.074+0.025, 0.067+0.024, and
0.086+0.026, respectively. This nucleotide diversity
indicates genetic variability of MHC genes both between and
within breeds.

8   Mapping of C2, Bf, and C4 Genes to the Swine Major
      Histocompatibility Complex (SLA) Wen-RONG LIE*, MAX F.
ROTHSCHILD, and CAROL M. WARNER Iowa State University, Ames, IA

Three miniature swine lines, inbred for SLA haplotypes, a,
c, and d, and a recombinant line, haplotype g, were analyzed for
possible restriction fragment length polymorphisms (RFLPs) by
Southern blot hybridization with human C2, factor B (Bf), and
C4 specific probes. The search for RFLPs by using a human C2
probe failed to reveal any variants. However, a TaqI polymorphism was identified with the human Bf probe and BamHI and PvuII
polymorphisms were identified with the human C4 probe. Overlapping restriction fragments were found with the C2 and Bf
probes, which strongly suggests close linkage of C2 and Bf genes
in swine. Segregation analyses of Bf and C4 polymorphisms indicated that polymorphic fragments followed a Mendelian pattern
of inheritance. The recombinant haplotype g, which expresses
class I genes of haplotype c and class II genes of haplotype d,
was shown to produce an identical RFLP pattern, using the Bf
and C4 probes, as haplotype d, but different from that of haplotype c. This indicates that there is a close association of
[C4-Bf-C2] and class II genes in miniature swine.

17   Characterization of B-F Molecules in the Chicken. KIMBERLY
      KLINE, W. ELWOOD BRILES, LARRY BACON, AND BOB G.
SANDERS* Dept. of Zoology, University of Texas, Austin, TX. 78712.

B-F alloantisera recognize distinct 45 Kd molecules on peripheral red blood
cells (RBC) from embryonic chickens and heterogeneous MW molecules of
approximately 40-44 Kd on peripheral RBC from adult chickens, provisionally
referred to as type 1 and type 2 molecules, respectively. Type 2 molecules have
a basic pI, exhibit multiple isomorphic variants, and are associated with a
smaller polypeptide of approximately 11-12 Kd assumed to be beta-2-
microglobulin. Type 1 molecules have an acidic pI, exhibit limited
heterogeneity, and are not associated with a smaller polypeptide. Type 1 and
type 2 molecules were also shown to be distinct by peptide mapping and
serological analyses. In addition, two distinct molecular weight forms of the
type 2 molecules were distinguished, provisionally referred to as 2A (45 Kd)
and 2B (42 Kd). In vivo-derived avian erythroblastosis virus (AEV)-
transformed erythroleukemia cells expressed type 2A molecules. In vitro cloned
AEV-transformed erythroleukemia cells expressed very low levels of B-F
molecules however, they expressed type 2B molecules when induced to
differentiate. Normal bursa-derived lymphoid cells expressed type 2A
molecules while normal thymus-derived lymphoid cells expressed type 2B
molecules. Cloned reticuloendotheliosis virus (REV)-transformed immature
lymphoid cells expressed either type 2A or 2B molecules.

18   Structural Studies on Chicken B-L Antigens Using
      Monoclonal Antibodies to Monomorphic Determinants.
JOHN M. BERESTECKY* and ALBERT A. BENEDICT, Department of
Microbiology, University of Hawaii, Honolulu, Hawaii 96822.

Four monoclonal antibodies (MAb), B1, B4, B10 and CIa-1
(Ewert,D.L. et al. J.I. 132:2524, 1984), reacted with non-
polymorphic determinants on chicken B-L antigens. Although
these MAb reacted with all chickens of numerous lines, their
reactions with peripheral blood lymphocytes of other bird
species differed. B1 reacted with all genera tested of the
family Phasianidae as well as with some genera outside of the
family. The distribution of the B4 and B10 epitopes differed
and neither was as widely represented as the B1 or the CIa-1
epitopes.
      B1 was used to specifically purify B-L antigen from lysates
of the RP9 cell line. The molecule resisted SDS denaturation
but was sensitive to moderate heat treatment in the absence of
SDS. Heating at 70°-80°C dissociated the molecule into heavy
and light polypeptide chains as identified by silver staining
and western blotting 2-D gels. The B1 epitope on the light
chain was resistant to further heating but was sensitive to
reduction. The B4, B10 and CIa-1 epitopes were found on the
affinity purified molecules but not on the dissociated chains.

19   Production and biochemical characterization of a mouse
      monoclonal antibody (MAb) detecting chicken MHC
                    class II (B-L) antigen

HYUN S. LILLEHOJ*, SAMUEL KIM AND ERIK P. LILLEHOJ. Animal
Parasitology Institute, ARS, USDA, Beltsville, MD, 20705,
Program Resources Inc., Frederick, MD. 21701

    A mouse monoclonal antibody (P3x2-1-1 MAb) that detects
chicken class II antigen was produced from the fusion of P3x
myeloma cells with spleen cells from BALB/C mice immunized
with chicken spleen. FACS analysis of P3x2-1-1 MAb staining
of lymphocytes from SC and FP chickens showed 80% staining
of the bursa, 15-20% staining of spleen cells and PBL and
less than 5% (background) staining of thymus cells.
Addition of the MAb to T cell ConA cultures showed slight
inhibition of T cell proliferation whereas removal of P3x2-
1-1 reactive cells prior to ConA stimulation did not
interfere with T cell activation. The MAb inhibited mixed
lymphocyte response of splenic T cells. SDS-PAGE analysis
of ^{35}S labelled spleen cells identified 28, 30, and 32 KD
antigens. This study shows that MAb P3x2-1-1 detects a
monomorphic determinant of the chicken class II antigen.

20   **Cell Surface Ia Expression on Chicken Inflammatory
      Macrophages**. RODNEY R. DIETERT* and KAREN A. GOLEMBOSKI.
Cornell University, Ithaca, NY 14853.

    Flow cytometry was used to compare the expression of cell
surface Ia on K-strain chicken inflammatory macrophages.
Macrophage Ia expression was compared with that of both bursal
lymphocytes and the transformed macrophage cell line, HD11. A
monoclonal antibody directed against a monomeric Ia epitope
(Southern Biotechnology) was used. Macrophage-rich peritoneal
exudate cells collected 4 hrs after i.p. Sephadex injection
exhibited a significantly reduced percentage of Ia-positive
cells compared with cells harvested 42 hrs after Sephadex
administration. Likewise, both the fluorescent intensity of
Ia-positive 4 hr cells and their size as measured by time of
flight were significantly reduced when compared with similar
parameters from 42 hr post-injection cells. Bursal lymphocytes
and HD11 macrophages had mean fluorescent intensities similar
to the levels found on 4 hr inflammatory macrophages. The
temporal shift in macrophage Ia expression during the early
stages of the inflammatory response is associated with changes
in the functional capacities of peritoneal macrophages.

21   Functional and biochemical analysis of a recombination between chicken
MHC class I and class II genes. OLLI VAINIO*, BRIGITTE RIWAR and OLLI
LASSILA, Basel Institute for Immunology, Basel, Switzerland.

Previous studies have already suggested that CB (B12/12) and H.B19 (B19/19)
chickens have different major histocompatibility complex (MHC) class I (B-F) and
erythrocyte-specific B-G gene products, whereas the class II (B-L) antigens seem
to be indistinguishable. The B-L12 and B-L19 antigen identity is supported by
the absence of specific alloantibody production after extensive cross immunization, complete cross-wise absorption of alloantibodies, weak graft-versus-host
and mixed lymphocyte reactions and by the ability of B-L12 and B-L19 antigens to
serve as identical restriction elements for T-B cell cooperation in antibody
production in vivo. Recently, it was also reported that B-L12 and B-L19 genes
have similar restriction fragment length polymorphism (RFLP) patterns as analyzed by genomic Southern hybridization with human class II β gene-specific probes. In the present study we show that B-L12 and B-L19 antigens are functionally
as efficient to present antigen (keyhole limpet hemocyanin, KLH) to B12/12 KLH-
specific T cell clone as measured by a T cell proliferation assay. Furthermore,
we demonstrate that anti B-L monoclonal antibody gives similar immunoprecipitation patterns from biosynthetically labelled B12/12 and B19/19 bursa cells as
analyzed by 2-dimensional gel electrophoresis. In conclusion, our present
results together with the earlier data strongly support the hypothesis that a
DNA recombination event has separated B-L from B-F and B-G.

22   AN ATTEMPT TO DETECT RECOMBINATION WITHIN THE CHICKEN MHC
BY MEANS OF MIXED LYMPHOCYTE REACTION.
K. HÀLA[1], O. LASSILA[2], and C. AUFFRAY[3]. [1]Inst. for Gen. & Exp.
Pathology, University of Innsbruck, Austria, [2]Basel Institute
for Immunology, Basel, Switzerland, [3]Institute of Embryology,
CNRS, Nogent sur Marne, France.

All recombinants so far described arose from recombination
between the B-L and B-G regions or within the B-G region. The
present experiments were undertaken to answer the question
whether recombinations exist between B-L and B-F. By serological methods, using monoclonal antibodies and alloantibodies,
no recombinants between these two loci (B-L and B-F) were found
among 1155 F2 and F3 birds from CB x CC crosses. About 1% of
the F2 birds gave abnormal mixed lymphocyte reactions. We are
currently analyzing these birds by progeny testing and by
restriction fragment length polymorphism with a B-L β DNA
probe.

Supported by the Austrian Cancer Research Fund.

23   Characterization of BoLA class II types by 1D - IEF.

IRMA JOOSTEN, BOUKE G. HEPKEMA and EVERT J. HENSEN*
Dept. of Immunology, Fac. of Veterinary Medicine, University of
Utrecht, P.O. Box 80.165 Utrecht, The Netherlands.

Typing for BoLA class II products, in contrast with typing
for HLA class II products, has not been successful till now. In
humans, one dimensional isoelectric focussing (IEF) of immunoprecipitates of class II products showed banding patterns which
correlated very well with typing by serology. It appeared possible to (sub)type on banding patterns.
For the characterization of BoLA products we used a crossreactive
rabbit antiserum raised against purified human class II antigens.
Bovine class II products were immunoprecipitated from detergent
extracts of biosynthetically radiolabeled peripheral blood lymphocytes. Immunoprecipitates were analysed by SDS-PAGE, 2D electro-
foresis (IEF/SDS-PAGE) and 1D-IEF. Molecular weights and IEF
characteristics of immunoprecipitates from cattle cells were
homologous to those of human class II products. In family studies
segregation of independent banding patterns was observed. Defined
sets of bands, as characterised in the segregation study, were
found in a panel of non-related animals.Currently, 1D-IEF is also
used for (sub)typing of BoLA classI products. This technique may
be of great help in the elucidation of MHC polymorphism in cattle
as well as in other species.

24   **2-Dimensional Electrophoretic Analysis of BoLA**
**THEODORE L. GARBER*, LAREE M. HUFFMAN, JOE W.
TEMPLETON. Texas A & M University,   Veterinary
Pathology Dept., College Station, Texas 77843.**

**Bovine class I major histocompatibility antigens
(BoLA) were immunoprecipitated from fresh or mitogen
stimulated peripheral blood lymphocytes using
monoclonal antibody W6/32 and biochemically analysed
by 2-dimensional (IEF & SDS-PAGE) gel electrophoresis.   Each BoLA serotype appears to be represented as a unique pattern of spots with animals
sharing BoLA specificities displaying   partially
superimposable gel fingerprints.   Treatment   of
immunoprecipitated antigens with neuraminidase is
necessary prior to electrophoresis to reduce the
complexity of the fingerprint. Transmission of   2-D
gel patterns within families is continuing to   be
studied to determine the number of BoLA class I
genes expressed on the bovine lymphocyte.**

25

<u>Identification of major histocompatibility complex HLA-DR-like and HLA-DQ-like loci products in a bovine lymphoblastoid cell line.</u>   ANNE M. JANZER-PFEIL* AND GARY A. SPLITTER.   Department of Veterinary Science, University of Wisconsin, Madison, WI 53706.

Bovine major histocompatibility complex (MHC) class II loci products were investigated using monoclonal antibodies (Mabs) with known MHC class II specificities in other species.   Mabs were tested for reactivity with the bovine lymphoblastoid cell line, BL3, using indirect fluorescent antibody labeling and analysis by flow cytometry.   Postitive Mabs were used to immunoprecipitate class II antigens from BL3 lysate labeled with ^{35}S-methionine and solubilized with NP40.   Immunoprecipitates were separated by sodium dodecyl sulfate polyacrylamide gel electrophoresis and visualized by autoradiography.

Mabs yielding successful immunoprecipitations and with known loci specificity in other species were then used in sequential immunoprecipitations.   HLA-DR specific Mab (H4) and HLA-DQ specific Mab (CC11.23) were used to identify the presence of both DR-like and DQ-like loci products in BL3 cell lysate.   Current work in our laboratory is focusing on two-dimensional gel electrophoresis to correlate with the sequential immunoprecipitations for a clearer understanding of the bovine MHC class II loci products.

26

<u>Isolation and Characterization of γ-ray Induced MHC Loss Mutants of a Bovine Lymphoblastoid Cell Line.</u>   JEROME S. HARMS* AND GARY A. SPLITTER, Department of Veterinary Science, University of Wisconsin, Madison, WI 53706

Using the monoclonal antibody WIM 8.1 and complement, seven BoLA Loss mutants were selected after γ-ray induced mutagenesis of the bovine lymphoblastoid cell line BL3.   WIM 8.1 had been shown through microcytotoxicity tests to be antigen specific for the BoLA class I allele w8 located also on the heterozygons class I (w8/w7) BL3 cell line.   After mutation and selection, the surviving fraction of cells were cloned and tested for true BoLA loss mutants using microcytotoxicity resulting in seven w8-antigen loss mutants of the parent BL3.

Further characterizations of the variants were done using flow cytometry with antibodies to class I and class II antigens.   Using the selecting antibody WIM 8.1, expected results followed; virtually no expression of w8 on any of the variants.   However, using the HLA class II antibodies H4 (DR specific) and CC11 (DQ specific), a marked decrease in expression of these class II antigens were observed in all the mutants to varying degrees.

Data from FACS analysis lead to functional and molecular studies now underway with the goal that characterization of these seven variants will help in understanding the major histocompatibility complex of the bovine system.

27   BOLA class II typing using interspecies crossreactive reagents and
      immunomagnetic spheres.

       1   1   1   2   3
      Ø.Lie, M.Syed*, I.Olsaker, F.Vartdal & J.Ugelstad.

      1. Dept. of Genetics and Biotechnical Disease Control.
      The Norwegian College of Veterinary Medicine & National Veterinary
      Institute, Oslo.

      2.Institute of Transplantation Immunology, National Hospital, Oslo.

      3. Institute of Industrial Chemestry, University of Trondheim.

Highly viable class II+ bovine cells have been isolated within 5 min
(after a 5 min incubation) from whole blood in a one step procedure.
This is achieved by magnetic seperation of rosettes formed between the
cells and superparamagnetic monosized polystyrene micropheres coated
with Mabs specific for HLA class II monomorphic epitopes.
Preliminary data show that even polymorphic HLA class II Mabs may be
used to identify BOLA class II specificities. Employing human B-chain
CDNA probes for DP,DQ and DR genes, we have by RFLP analysis demonstrated polymorphism in all three corresponding subregions of B-chain.

28   Genetic Markers for Detecting Major Genes for Quantitative
      Traits: Segregation of BoLA Haplotypes in Paternal Half-
sibs. JONATHAN E. BEEVER*, JULIE A. STEWART, HARRIS A. LEWIN,
and PHILLIP D. GEORGE.   Department   of Animal Sciences,
University of Illinois, Urbana, IL.   61801.

Genetic markers may be used in the future as a tool for
genetic improvement of domestic animals. It is our objective to
use the BoLA-A locus and six other informative polymorphic
genetic loci as genetic markers to detect major genes for growth
and carcass composition in beef cattle.   To date 112 paternal
half-sibs have been genotyped at the BoLA-A(class I) locus using
a panel of serological reagents that identify allelic products
of the bovine MHC. Identification of each segregating haplotype
was performed with parous antisera which had pairwise r-values
of not less than .60.   The two haplotypes were marked by the
class I alleles W2 and UR28.   Segregation tended to favor the
W2 bearing haplotype (p<.10), with 66 of the half-sibs
inheriting the W2 allele and 46 inheriting the UR28 allele. The
effect of BoLA haplotype and other marker bearing chromosomes on
birth, 205-day, weaning, and yearling weights and carcass
composition is currently in progress. (Work supported by USDA
Grant #87-CRCR-1-2292)

29   Characterization of Monoclonal Antibodies (mAb) Reactive
      with Swine Major Histocompatibility Complex (MHC or SLA)
Antigens. DIANA IVANOSKA, DONALD C. SUN*, and JOAN K. LUNNEY.
Animal Parasitology Institute, Agricultural Research Service,
USDA, Beltsville, MD 20705 and INEP, Zemun, Yugoslavia.

MAb reactive with allodeterminants of SLA antigens have been
produced from BALB/c mice immunized with PBL from SLA inbred
miniature swine. Hybridoma supernatants were characterized by
their reactivity with PBL from SLA d/d(dd), cc, and aa swine,
and by the mw of the antigen precipitated from ^{35}S methionine
labeled PBL. Use of SLA class I gene transfected L cells (D.S.
Singer et al., PNAS 79 1403,1982) enabled us to prove that some
mAb differentially reacted with SLA class I gene products. MAb
reactive with SLA class I gene products include: 2.27.3, IgG_1,
reactive with all swine PBL and binding L cells transfected with
either PD1 or PD14 SLA class I genes; 2.28.1, IgM, reactive with
all swine PBL but binding only to cells transfected with PD1 DNA;
2.32.1, IgG, and 2.12.3, IgM, reactive with dd PBL, nonreactive
with aa or cc PBL, and binding only to PD14 transfected L cells.
These mAb will be useful for future studies of viral T cell
reactivity and of SLA gene expression in SLA transgenic animals.
Currently, attempts are being made to produce additional mAb
against allodeterminants of swine class II MHC antigens.

30   Ten Serologically-Defined Lymphocyte Alloantigens
      Identified in North American Pigs
MING-CHE WU*, YUN-CHAO SHIA, DAVID G. MCLAREN, HARRIS A.
LEWIN and LAWRENCE B. SCHOOK. Dept. of Animal Sciences,
University of Illinois, Urbana 61801, USA.

A new panel of serological reagents that identifies putative allelic products of swine major histocompatibility complex (SLA) was developed. Using the lymphocyte microcytotoxicity test, a total of 191 parous sera were screened
and selected against 28 random cells and 36 paternal half
sib crossbred gilts. The computer programs CLUSTER and
SERAGRAF were used to identify ten clusters of sera designated as UR1, UR2, UR3, UR4, UR4.1, UR5, UR6, UR7, UR8 and
UR9. Segregation analysis indicated that specificities UR1
and UR2 were allelic with allelism correlation of -.55
(P<.001). These reagents are the first produced for SLA-
typing of outbred pigs in the United States. Additional
families are being studied for further serological and
molecular characterization of the SLA complex. (Supported
by a grant from the National Pork Producers' Council).

31   Title: "MAJOR HISTOCOMPATIBILITY COMPLEX IN SHEEP (OLA).
              1. Genetic control of lymphocyte antigens detec-
ted by sera produced in Spanish Merino Sheep".

Authors: ARGERICH, Mª Cristina & LLANES, Diego*

Address: Departamento de Genetica. Instituto de Zootecnia. Fa-
         cultad de Veterinaria. Universidad de Cordoba. SPAIN.

Sera from 122 Merino sheep were screened for citotoxic antibodies against sheep lymphocytes. Twenty sera were selected --
which provisionally define 6 lymphocyte antigens named SM1,
SM2, SM3, SM4, SM5 and SM6. Family studies show that   inheritance of these sheep lymphocyte specificities is controled by
autosomal codominant genes. Our results are consistent with
the hipothesis of at least 2 linked loci. We have compared SM
antigens with previous reported by P. Millot and some although
weakly correlations have been found.

32   Serological Definition of the Major Histocompatibility
       Complex in the Domestic Cat. [1]CHERYL A. WINKLER*, [2]ALLEN
SCHULTZ, and [3]STEPHEN J. O'BRIEN, [1]Program Resources, Inc.,
[2]BRI, [3]NCI, Frederick Cancer Research Facility, Frederick,
Maryland 21701-1013

Skin allografts were exchanged between cats to determine the
extent of MHC polymorphism and to raise lymphocytotoxic alloantisera against MHC antigens. Evidence for MHC polymorphism
comes from the observation that 25% of the allografts between
sibs had prolonged survival while all allografts between
unrelated or parent-offspring pairs were rapidly rejected.
Thirteen lymphocytotoxic alloantisera specific for donor cells
were produced and tested on a panel of outbred cats. Association analysis identified six clusters of overlapping
antigenicities that were transmitted vertically in cat families.
Evidence that the lymphocytotoxic alloantisera are recognizing
MHC antigens is provided by increased survival time of skin
grafts between MHC identical sibs as compared to haplodistinct
or haploidentical sibs. Eight of the alloantisera immunoprecipitated class I glycoproteins and two immunoprecipitated class
II glycoproteins. Three of the alloantisera reacted with both
classes. The MHC of the cat has been named FLA and at least
three class I loci and one class II locus have been identified.

33 <u>Identification of the Major Histocompatibility Complex in</u>
<u>the Ring-necked Pheasant.</u> Susan I. Jarvi* and W.E. Briles.
Department of Biological Sciences, Northern Illinois University,
DeKalb, IL 60115 U.S.A.

A blood group system has been detected in the ring-necked
pheasant (<u>Phasianus colchicus</u>). A pair of pheasants were mated
and produced 13 progeny. Reciprocal immunizations between the
pair resulted in two antisera, each detecting specific antigens
transmitted by the donor to its progeny. Antigens transmitted
by the sire were tentatively designated A and B, and those
transmitted by the dam as C and D. Immunization between
selected sibs resulted in the production of antisera for the
specific detection of A, C or D. A panel of chicken reagents
specific for antigens of <u>A</u>, <u>B-F</u> and <u>B-G</u> demonstrated differential
reactivity of the cells of individual pheasants, which indicates
the presence of equivalent systems in this species. Reagents of
the "ABCD" system were demonstrated by indirect immunofluorescent
technique to also be reactive with lymphocyte surface antigens.
Data from hemagglutination, indirect immunofluorescent testing
of lymphocytes, and preliminary mixed lymphocyte reactions
indicate that these antigens represent haplotypes of the major
histocompatibility complex of the pheasant.

34 <u>Development of 15I$_5$-B Congenic Lines of Chickens.</u>
LARRY D. BACON* USDA-ARS-Regional Poultry Research
Laboratory, 3606 East Mount Hope Rd., East Lansing, Michigan
48823

Seven MHC (<u>B</u>)-types were introduced from other lines by F_1
matings to the histocompatible highly inbred line 15I$_5$. All
lines were inbred or selected for differences in susceptiblity
to viral induced leukosis or Marek's disease tumors. Initial
results of immunological and disease resistance traits for <u>B</u>-
homozygotes studied after 4-5 backcross generations will be
summarized. <u>B</u>-homozygotes maintained in a specific pathogen-
free environment are now being produced after 10 backcross
generations. Additional immunological, disease resistance, and
reproductive fitness studies are planned, as well as molecular
studies of MHC gene structure and expression.

35   The Effect of Genetic Selection on the Functional Capacity
        of the Immune System of Broilers.
                Z. Uni and E.D. Heller
        Faculty of Agriculture, P.O.B.12 REHOVOT 76100,   ISRAEL

Genetic selection for early immune responsiveness of a hetero-
genic population of broiler chickens was performed against two
antigens simultaneously, heat killed E.coli and Newcastle Disease
vaccine (NDV). The immune response was measured at young age, 14-
18 days. The chicks were divided into two populations according to
their responses: a population of high responders to both antigens
and a population of low or none responders.
After 4 generations of selection, a significant difference was
observed in the immune responses of the two populations. In
addition the two populations differed in their PBL binding of BNA,
the high responders showed lower number of BNA binding lymphocytes.
During the selection a segregation of MHC genes occured, the high
responder exhibited a high percentage of the B^5 genotype while the
low responders exhibited a high percentage of the B^{15} and B^{19}
genotypes.

36   *Bovine Lymphocytotropic Protozoan Theileria annulata:
        in vitro Culture Studies*

A.S.Grewal; A.P.Mangat; A.Singh & V.Bhattacharyulu
Tick Borne Diseases Research Centre,Punjab Agricultural University, Ludhiana-141 004, India.*

*Cultivation of T. annulata infected lymphocytes and
their use as live attenuated vaccine have been reported by various workers. Actively dividing infected
lymphocytes especially in primary culture phase were
vulnerable to heat labile component (56°,30') of
serum used in culture medium. This suggests possibility of complement activation by transformed lymphocytes. Presence of intralymphocyte schizonts and
intraerythrocyte piroplasms in smears from lymphoid
tissue biopsy and blood is conventional diagnostic
test of patent infections. In-vitro culture of
lymphocytes from experimental calves which did not
exhibit patent infections by these laboratory tests,
frequently developed intralymphocyte schizonts. We
find this culture method could also be a useful
sensitive diagnostic aid in clinical,epidemiological
studies and monitoring vaccine/chemotherapeutic
trials.*

37   Influence of the Porcine Major Histocompatibility Genes
      on Immune Response.
BONNIE A. MALLARD[*] AND BRUCE N. WILKIE, Dept. of Vet. Micro.
and Immunology, BRIAN KENNEDY, Dept. of Animal and Poultry
Science, University of Guelph, Guelph, Ontario, Canada, N1G 2W1.

Immune response was determined for three SLA-defined strains
of miniature swine (SLA^a, SLA^c, SLA^d) and one (ABC^{c}D^d)
recombinant strain (SLA^g).   Immunization was by a standard
protocol using antigens chosen for their known MHC-associated
immunogenicity and specific immunogenic properties. Analysis
of variance was by least squares on data from 133 pigs from 34
litters by 15 sires and 18 dams. The general linear model
accounted for the effects of SLA haplotype, sire, dam, sex of
pig and litter for each antigen examined. Results indicated
that SLA haplotype and dam effects significantly influenced the
skinfold thickness response to DNCB and PPD. Haplotype also
significantly influenced the primary and secondary serum
antibody response to sheep erythrocytes, and the synthetic
polypeptide (T,G)AL, as did non-MHC sire and dam factors.
Haplotype contributed significantly to the primary antibody
response to lysozyme as did other sire, dam and litter effects.

38   Effect of SLA Haplotype on Preimplantation Embryonic Development
      in Miniature Swine. NANCY K. SCHWARTZ*, ALAN J.CONLEY, MAX F.
ROTHSCHILD, CAROL M. WARNER and STEPHEN P. FORD. Depts. of Biochem.
Biophys. and Anim. Sci., Iowa State Univ., Ames, IA 50011.

Previous research from our laboratory, utilizing 3 strains of miniature swine bred for specific SLA haplotypes (a, c and d), demonstrated
that litters from either sows or boars with the d haplotype were larger than for all other matings. It has been hypothesized that the rate
of preimplantation embryonic development in the pig is associated with
survival to term. The aim was to compare the number of blastomeres per
embryo from SLA$^{a/a}$, SLA$^{c/c}$ and SLA$^{d/d}$ matings on day 6 postmating (day
0 = first day of mating) by nuclear staining and days 9 and 11 by DNA
analyses. Embryo numbers were greater for SLA$^{d/d}$ females than SLA$^{a/a}$
or SLA$^{c/c}$ (8.8 vs 6.8 and 6.2), while recovery rates (embryos recov-
ered/corpora lutea number) were similar, averaging 70.8, 74.4 and
73.2%, respectively. Embryos from SLA$^{d/d}$ females were less advanced in
development on day 6 than embryos from SLA$^{a/a}$ or SLA$^{c/c}$ which did not
differ (23 vs 89 and 79 blastomeres). The reduced cell numbers of
SLA$^{d/d}$ vs SLA$^{a/a}$ or SLA$^{c/c}$ embryos continued to day 9 (23 vs 107 and 67
ng DNA/embryo) and day 11 (167 vs 674 and 586 ng DNA/ embryo). These
data suggest an effect of the SLA complex on preimplantation embryonic
development.

39   Chicken B-F, B-G and β₂M cDNA clones. KARSTEN SKJOEDT*, ROLF ANDERSEN
        and JIM KAUFMAN, Institute for Experimental Immunology, Copenhagen,
        Denmark and Basel Institute for Immunology, Basel, Switzerland.
We constructed λgt11 cDNA libraries using spleen and bone marrow polyA⁺ RNA
from anemic B19 chickens. By screening with degenerate oligonucleotide probes,
we isolated a cDNA lacking only a portion pf the 3' UT, which when translated
matches the known chicken β₂M protein sequence exactly. We also isolated 3
putative BF and 9 putative BG cDNA clones by first screening with rabbit antisera to highly purified BG13 and GF15 and then testing induced positive clones
by absorbtion of sera, elution and Western blotting using red blood cell lysa-
tes. The 5' in-frame sequence of one 1400 bp BF clone (F3) has 35% amino
acid/60% nucleotide homology with mammalian class I exons 1 and 2. The BG clones range from 450-1400 bp, with some clones homologous at the 5' end. The BF
clone F3 and two anti-BG selected clones (G3 and G4, noncrosshybridizing) were
used to Southern blot DNA from various chicken strains including congenic and
recombinant lines. F3, G3 and G4 show polymorphic patterns with a numnber of
restriction enzymes which exactly correlated with MHC haplotype. F3 shows different and simpler patterns than G3 and G4, which have more bands including
some in common. G3 and G4 also show variation with more enzymes and more
strains than F3. These probes can be useful typing reagents, particularly for
uncharacterized chicken strains.

40   Pierre MILLOT - The Sheep OLA Complex

The sheep M.H.C. (OLA) includes 3 linked loci OLA-A, B and C
coding for 16 OLA factors; 14 of them are genetically defined
and distributed into 3 allelic series of 6, 5 and 3 factors.
2 other lymphocyte factors depend on 2 non OLA loci, of which
the first OL-X is loosely linked to OLA and the second OL-Z
independent of the Complex. The 3 OLA loci were in linkage
disequilibrium in a "Préalpe" flock; 28 haplotypes were
registered. A comparison test between some reagents was performed by P. CULLEN during 1983. A linkage between the OLA loci
and one sheep resistance/susceptibility locus to Scrapie (Scr)
was shown in 1985 and 1987 by statistical and family studies.
The recombination rate was estimated to be between 11 and
16%. Bent-Limb disease in lambs is linked to both the OL-Z
minor lymphocyte locus (independent of OLA) and the I locus
(controlling the epression of R/O blood groups antigens in
sheep).

Don Adams
Veterinary Anatomy
College of Vet. Med.
Iowa State University
Ames, Iowa 50011

Gerard A. Albers
Euribrid
P.O. Box 30
Boxmeer 5830 AA
THE NETHERLANDS

Darrilyn G. Albright
Veterinary Science Department
University of Kentucky
Lexington, KY 40546-0099

Cathy Almquist
Immunobiology
Iowa State University
Ames, Iowa 50011

Leif Andersson
Department of Animal Breeding
    and Genetics
Swedish University
Uppsala Biomedical Center, Box 596
S-751 24 Uppsala SWEDEN

Larry Arp
Veterinary Pathology
2720 Veterinary Medicine
Iowa State University
Ames, Iowa 50011

James A. Arthur
Hy-Line International
1915 Sugar Grove
Dallas Center, Iowa 50063

Charles Auffray
CNRS Et College De France
Institut D'Embryologie,
49 bis
94736 Nogent FRANCE

Larry D. Bacon
USDA-ARS Reg. Poultry
Res. Lab.
3606 East Mount Hope Rd.
East Lansing, MI 48823

Ernest F. Bailey
Department of Veterinary Science
University of Kentucky
Lexington, Kentucky 40506

T. R. Batra
Agriculture Canada
Animal Research Centre
Ottawa, Ontario
CANADA

Jonathan E. Beever
University of Illinois
114 ASL, 1207 W. Gregory
Urbana, IL 61801

Don Beitz
Animal Science
313 Kildee Hall
Iowa State University
Ames, Iowa 50011

T. K. Bell
Department of Physiology & Pharmacology
University of Queensland
St. Lucia Brisbane Queensland
AUSTRALIA 4067

John M. Berestecky
Department of Microbiology
University of Hawaii
101 Snyder Hall
Honolulu, Hawaii 96822

Han J. Blankert
Agricultural University
Department of Animal Husbandry
Marijkeweg 40
6709 PG Wageningen
THE NETHERLANDS

Stephen E. Bloom
Cornell University
215 Rice Hall
Department of Poultry & Avian Sciences
Ithaca, New York 14853

Sandra E. Bradley
RLH U.S. Meat Animal Research Center
Box 166
Clay Center, NE 68933

183

George Brant
119 Kildee Hall
Iowa State University
Ames, Iowa 50011

W. E. Briles
Biological Sciences
Northern Illinois University
DeKalb, IL 60115

Melody Brownell
Biochemistry Department
335B Gilman Hall
Iowa State University
Ames, Iowa 50011

Dennis Byrne
Department of Botany
353 Bessey Hall
Ames, Iowa 50011

Robert W. Bull
Department of Medicine
B220 Life Sciences Bldg.
Michigan State University
East Lansing, MI 48824

N. Bumstead
Houghton Poultry Research Station
St. Ives
Cambridgeshire
PE17 2DA ENGLAND

Sam Buttram
Department of Animal Breeding
239 Kildee Hall
Iowa State University
Ames, Iowa 50011

Victoria E. Carr
Microbiology
2823 West Street, #4
Ames, Iowa 50010

Patrick Chardon
Lab. de Radiobiologie Appliquée
CEA-IPSN, CRZ
Jouy-En-Josas FRANCE

Shen Cheng
Department of Animal Science
201 Kildee Hall
Iowa State University
Ames, Iowa 50011

Dr. Frank L. Cherms
Nicholas Turkey Breeding Farms
P.O. Box Y
Sonoma, CA 95476-1209

Lauren L. Christian
Department of Animal Science
119 Kildee Hall
Iowa State University
Ames, Iowa 50011

Larry V. Cundiff
USDA-ARS, Roman L. Hruska
U.S. Meat Animal Research Center
P.O. Box 166
Clay Center, NE 68933

George N. Daniels
Veterinary Pathology/Diagnostic Lab.
1655 Vet. Med.
Iowa State University
Ames, Iowa 50011

Chella David
Department of Immunology
Mayo Clinic and Medical School
Rochester, MN 55905

Christopher J. Davies
USDA-ARS Animal Parasitology Institute
Building 1040 Room 2
BARC-East
Beltsville, MD 20705

Mary DeBey
Vet. Micro.
Iowa State University
Ames, Iowa 50011

Edward V. Deverson
Department of Immunology
Institute of Animal Physiology & Genetics
     Research
Babraham Hall, Babraham Cambridge CB2 4AT
UNITED KINGDOM

John R. Diehl
Animal Science
Clemson University
Clemson, SC 29634-0361

Rodney R. Dietert
Poultry and Avian Sciences
216 Rice Hall
Cornell University
Ithaca, New York 14853

Peggy Dillender
University of Iowa
Department of Microbiology
Bowen Science Building
Iowa City, Iowa 52242

Michael P. Dooley
Veterinary Physiology & Pharmacology
College of Vet. Med.
Iowa State University
Ames, Iowa 50011

Donald D. Draper
Vet. Anatomy
1062 Vet. Med.
Iowa State University
Ames, Iowa 50011

Edith R. Erkert
Northern Illinois University
Department of Biological Sciences
DeKalb, Illinois 60115-2861

Deborah L. Fairchild
Immunogenetics Laboratory
Ohio State University
2027 Coffey Road
Columbus, Ohio 43210

Jane Fagerland
Department of Vet. Pathology
Iowa State University
Ames, Iowa 50011

Walter Fehr
Office of Biotechnology
11301 Agronomy
Iowa State University
Ames, Iowa 50011

Cindy Fitch-Steenson
Genetics
8 Curtiss
Iowa State University
Ames, Iowa 50011

Mike Flanagan
Biochemistry Department
325 Gilman Hall
Iowa State University
Ames, Iowa 50011

S. P. Ford
Department of Animal Science
11 Kildee Hall
Iowa State University
Ames, Iowa 50011

A. E. Freeman
Department of Animal Science
239 Kildee Hall
Iowa State University
Ames, Iowa 50011

John C. Fuller, Jr.
Animal Science
156 Food Tech.
Iowa State University
Ames, Iowa 50011

Janet E. Fulton
Department of Animal Science
201 Kildee Hall
Iowa State University
Ames, Iowa 50011

Theodore L. Garber
Texas A & M University
Veterinary Pathology Department
College Station, TX 77843

Catherine Gautschi
Institute fur Tierzucht
University of Berne
Bremgartenstr. 109a
CH-3012 Berne
SWITZERLAND

John Gerlach
Department of Medicine
B220 Life Sciences Building
Michigan State University
East Lansing, Michigan 48824

Brad Gerndt
Biochemistry Department
335B Gilman Hall
Iowa State University
Ames, Iowa 50011

Anne R. Greenlee
Department of Vet. Micro. Path.
Washington State University
402 Bustad Vet. Sci. Bldg.
Pullman, WA 99164-7040

A. S. Grewal
Tick Borne Disease Research Centre
College of Veterinary Sciences
Ludhiana-141 004
INDIA

Gerard Guerin
Laboratoire de Genetique biochimique
INRA-CRJ
78350 Jouy-en-Josas
FRANCE

Karel Hála
Institute for General & Experimental Path.
University of Innsbruck
Fritz-Pregl-Strasse 3
A-6020 Innsbruck
AUSTRIA

Vickie Hall
Biochemistry Department
397 Gilman Hall
Iowa State University
Ames, Iowa 50011

Richard Hamilton
Department of Zoology
Science II
Iowa State University
Ames, Iowa 50011

David J. Hannapel
Horticulture
Iowa State University
Ames, Iowa 50011

Susan Harlocker
Department of Zoology
539 Science II Building
Iowa State University
Ames, Iowa 50011

Jerome S. Harms
University of Wisconsin
1655 Linden Drive
Madison, WI 53706

James A. Harp
National Animal Disease Center
P.O. Box 70
Ames, Iowa 50010

D. L. Harris
Pig Improvement Co.
Rural Route 1
P.O. Box 65
Rothville, MO 64676

I. T. Harris
Pig Improvement Co.
Rural Route 1
P.O. Box 65
Rothville, MO 64676

Nancy Harvey
Biochemistry Department
335G Gilman Hall
Iowa State University
Ames, Iowa 50011

David Harwood
Campbell Institute for Research &
Technology
POB 179
Farmington, AR 72730

Robert J. Hasiak
Animal Science
201 Kildee Hall
Iowa State University
Ames, Iowa 50011

Lanoy N. Hazel
Route 3 Box 227
Mountain Home, AR 72653

Dan E. Heller
Department of Animal Science
Faculty of Agriculture
P.O.B. 12
Rehovot 76100 ISRAEL

Dianne Hellwig
Vet. Pathology
Iowa State University
Ames, Iowa 50011

Suzanne Hendrich
Food and Nutrition
34 MacKay Hall
Iowa State University
Ames, Iowa 50011

Evert J. Hensen
Department of Immunology
Fac. Vet. Med.
University Utrecht
P.O. Box 80.165
Utrecht, THE NETHERLANDS

Bouke G. Hepkema
Department of Immunology
University Utrecht
P.O. Box 80.165
Utrecht, THE NETHERLANDS

H. C. Hines
Immunogenetics Laboratory
Ohio State University
2027 Coffey Road
Columbus, Ohio 43210

M. Peter Hoffman
119 Kildee Hall
Iowa State University
Ames, Iowa 50011

Andrew Holliman
Animal Health Trust
Balaton Lodge, Snailwell Road
Newmarket, Suffolk CB8 7DW
UNITED KINGDOM

Dennis Hulme
Department of Animal Husbandry
University of Sydney
NSW, 2006
AUSTRALIA

Diane Janick-Buckner
Gilman Hall
Biochemistry Department
Iowa State University
Ames, Iowa 50011

Anne M. Janzer-Pfeil
University of Wisconsin
1655 Linden Drive
Madison, Wisconsin 53706

Susan I. Jarvi
Biological Sciences
Northern Illinois University
DeKalb, Illinois 60115

Karalee Jarvill
VMRI
Iowa State University
Ames, Iowa 50011

Joseph T. Jensen
Diamond Scientific Co.
2538 SE 43rd Street
Des Moines, Iowa 50302

Kristine Johansen
VMRI
Iowa State University
Ames, Iowa 50011

Tom S. Johnson
Department of Biochemistry
B417 Agronomy
Iowa State University
Ames, Iowa 50011

Young Chul Jung
Department of Animal Science
233 Kildee Hall
Iowa State University
Ames, Iowa 50011

Michael Kaiser
Department of Animal Science
201 Kildee Hall
Iowa State University
Ames, Iowa 50011

Barry J. Kelly
Nicholas Turkey Breeding Farms
P.O. Box Y
Sonoma, CA 95476-1209

Chong Dae Kim
Department of Animal Science
201 Kildee Hall
Iowa State University
Ames, Iowa 50011

Kimberly Kline
Division of Nutrition
Department of Home Economics
University of Texas-Austin
Austin, Texas 78712

Kevin Knudtson
VMRI
Iowa State University
Ames, Iowa 50011

Ted Kramer
Vet. Microbiology
Iowa State University
Ames, Iowa 50011

Dan Kroll
Genetics Student
712 Clark
Ames, Iowa 50010

Al Kulenkamp
Shaver Poultry Breeding Farms, Ltd.
37 Randall Road
Cambridge, Ontario N3C 1R8
CANADA

Warren C. Ladiges
Division of Animal Medicine SB-42
University of Washington
Seattle, WA 98195

George Lambert
National Animal Disease Center, USDA-ARS
P.O. Box 70
Ames, Iowa 50010

Susan J. Lamont
Department of Animal Science
201 Kildee Hall
Iowa State University
Ames, Iowa 50011

Carol J. Landers
Biochemistry Department
Gilman Hall
Iowa State University
Ames, Iowa 50011

Ray A. Larsen
Department of Vet. Microbiology
Washington State University
Pullman, Washington 99614

Sandor Lazary
Institute for Animal Breeding, Berne
Bremgartenster 109
CH-3012 Berne
SWITZERLAND

H. W. Leipold
Department of Pathology
Kansas State University
Manhattan, Kansas 66506

Harris A. Lewin
Department of Animal Science
University of Illinois
114 ASL 1207 West Gregory Drive
Urbana, Illinois 61820

Wumin Li
University of Wisconsin
1655 Linden Drive
Madison, WI 53706

Wen-Rong Lie
Department of Biochemistry & Biophysics
325 Gilman Hall
Iowa State University
Ames, Iowa 50011

Hyun S. Lillehoj
Animal Parasitology Institute
U.S. Department of Agriculture
BARC-East Building 1040
Beltsville, MD 20705

Ruiz D. Llanes
Genetica. Universidad de Cordoba
Facultad de Veterinaria Avda Medina Azahara
Universidad de Cordoba, Cordoba 14005 SPAIN

Joan Lunney
USDA, Animal Parasitology Institute
Building 1040 BARC-East
Beltsville, MD 20705

Greg Mahairas
VMRI
Iowa State University
Ames, Iowa 50011

Bonnie Mallard
Department of Vet. Micro & Immunology
University of Guelph
Guelph, Ontario
CANADA N1G 2W1

Paul A. Martin
Vet. Med.
Iowa State University
Ames, Iowa 50011

Michael D. McFarland
Diamond Scientific Co.
2538 SE 43rd Street
Des Moines, Iowa 50317

David G. McLaren
University of Illinois
126 Animal Sciences Lab.
1207 W. Gregory Drive
Urbana, IL 61801

David Meeker
National Pork Producers Council
Box 10383
Des Moines, Iowa 50306

Marcia M. Miller
Beckman Research Institue
Department of Molecular Biochemistry
1450 E. Duarte Road
Duarte, CA 91010

Timothy J. Miller
Animal Health - Molecular Genetics
SmithKline & French Labs.
P.O. Box 1539
King of Prussia, PA 19406-0939

Wilmer J. Miller
Genetics Department
Iowa State University
Ames, Iowa 50011

F. Chris Minion
Vet. Med.
Iowa State University
Ames, Iowa 50011

Sowmya Moorthi
Genetics
240 Science II
Iowa State University
Ames, Iowa 50011

Donald O. Morgan
USDA, ARS, NAA, PIADC
P.O. Box 848
Greenport, NY 11944

Noelle E. Muggli
USDA, ARS, Roman L. Hruska
U.S. Meat Animal Research Center
P.O. Box 166
Clay Center, NE 68933-0166

Rosalee S. Muschott
Immunogenetics Laboratory
Ohio State University
2027 Coffey Road
Columbus, Ohio 43210

Mark J. Newman
Veterinary Microbiology
School of Vet. Med.
Louisiana State University
Baton Rouge, LA 70803

Marit Nilsen-Hamilton
MCDB & Biochemistry
A304 Gilman Hall
Iowa State University
Ames, Iowa 50011

A. W. Nordskog
Department of Animal Science
201 Kildee Hall
Iowa State University
Ames, Iowa 50011

Pierre Paré
Department of Animal Science
201 Kildee Hall
Iowa State University
Ames, Iowa 50011

Carol A. Park
Immunogenetics Laboratory
Ohio State University
2027 Coffey Road
Columbus, Ohio 43210

Peter A. Peterson
Department of Agronomy
Iowa State University
Ames, Iowa 50011

Carl A. Pinkert
Department of Animal Science
University of Missouri
164 Animal Sciences Center
Columbia, MO 65211

Jacob Pitcovski
Biochemistry Department
Gilman Hall
Iowa State University
Ames, Iowa 50011

Anthony Pusateri
Department of Animal Science
11 Kildee Hall
Iowa State University
Ames, Iowa 50011

Muquarrab A. Qureshi
Poultry Science
North Carolina State University
Raleigh, NC 27695

Tom Rehberger
Food Technology
210 Dairy Industry Building
Ames, Iowa 50011

Misi Robinson
USDA, ARS, Roman L. Hruska
U.S. Meat Animal Reserach Center
P.O. Box 166
Clay Center, NE 68933-0166

Mike Roof
Department of. Vet. Micro
Iowa State University
Ames, Iowa 50011

R. Rosenbusch
VMRI
Iowa State University
Ames, Iowa 50011

Martha Jane Ross
Immunogenetics Laboratory
Ohio State University
2027 Coffey Road
Columbus, Ohio 43210

James A. Roth
Department of Veterinary Microbiology
Iowa State University
Ames, Iowa 50011

Max F. Rothschild
Department of Animal Science
225 Kildee Hall
Iowa State University
Ames, Iowa 50011

Thora J. Runyan
Food and Nutrition
Iowa State University
Ames, Iowa 50011

David Sachs
Immunology Branch, NCI
National Institute of Health
Building 10, Room 4B17
Bethesda, MD 20205

Bob G. Sanders
Department of Zoology
University of Texas-Austin
Austin, Texas 78712

Ulla M. Sarmiento
Fred Hutchinson Cancer Research Centre
1124 Columbia Street
Seattle, WA 98104

Hal I. Sellers
Farmers Hybrid Co., Inc.
P.O. Box 4528
Des Moines, Iowa 50306

Mary Jo F. Schmeer
National Animal Disease Center
P.O. Box 70
Ames, Iowa 50010

Sheila Schmutz
Department of Veterinary Anatomy
University of Saskatchewan
Saskatoon, CANADA

Lawrence B. Schook
Animal Sciences
315 Animal Sciences Laboratory
1207 West Gregory Drive
Urbana, Illinois 61801

Nancy K. Schwartz
Biochemistry Department
325 Gilman Hall
Iowa State University
Ames, Iowa 50011

Joe Sebranek
Animal Science
215 Meat Lab
Iowa State University
Ames, Iowa 50011

Yun-Chao Shia
Animal Sciences
315 Sciences Laboratory
1207 West Gregory Drive
Urbana, Illinois 61801

Frank A. Simmen
Department of Animal Science & Laboratories
Ohio Agricultural Research & Development
Center
Ohio State University
Wooster, Ohio 44691

Dinah Singer
Immunology Branch, NCI
National Institute of Health
Building 10
Bethesda, MD 20205

Michele K. Smart
Biochemistry
B417 Agronomy
Iowa State University
Ames, Iowa 50011

Philip L. Spike
Department of Animal Science
225 Kildee Hall
Iowa State University
Ames, Iowa 50011

Gary A. Splitter
University of Wisconsin
1655 Linden Drive
Madison, WI 53706

Roger L. Spooner
Animal Breeding Research Center
West Mains Road
Edinburgh EH93JQ SCOTLAND

Miroslaw Stankiewicz
Vet. Med.
Iowa State University
Ames, Iowa 50011

Edward Steadham
Department of Animal Science
201 Kildee Hall
Iowa State University
Ames, Iowa 50011

Michael J. Stear
RLH U.S. Meat Animal Research Center
Box 166
Clay Center, Nebraska 68933

Emmett Stevermer
Animal Science
109 Kildee Hall
Iowa State University
Ames, Iowa 50011

Julie A. Stewart
Department of Animal Science
University of Illinois
1207 West Gregory
Urbana, Illinois 61801

Roger T. Stone
USDA, ARS Roman L. Hruska
U.S. Meat Animal Research Center
P.O. Box 166
Clay Center, NE 68933-0166

Donald Sun
USDA, Animal Parasitology Institute
Building 1040 BARC-East
Beltsville, MD 20705

Aree Sung
Biochemistry Department
Gilman Hall
Iowa State University
Ames, Iowa 50011

Mohasina Syed
Department of Biological Sciences
Stanford University
Stanford, CA 94305-5020

Michael J. Taylor
Vet. Physiology & Pharmacology
Iowa State University
Ames, Iowa 50011

Joe Templeton
Veterinary Pathology Department
Texas A & M University
College Station, TX 77843

Mark Teutsch
Department of Animal Science
University of Illinois
114 ASL
1207 Gregory Drive
Urbana, IL 61801

Marcel G.J. Tilanus
Agricultural University
Department of Exp. Animal Morph. and Cell
Biology
Marijkeweg 40
6709 PG, Wageningen, THE NETHERLANDS

Leo Timms
Animal Science
4 Kildee Hall
Iowa State University
Ames, Iowa 50011

Richard Towner
H & N International
15305 NE 40th Street
Redmond, WA 98052

Z. Uni
Department of Animal Science
Faculty of Agriculture
P.O.B. 12
Rehovot 76100 ISRAEL

Marcel Vaiman
IPSN-Departement de Protection Sanitaire
L.R.A. 91191 Gif Sur Yvette Cedex
Gif Sur Yvette 91191
FRANCE

Olli Vainio
Basel Institute for Immunology
Postfach
Grenzcherstrasse 487
SWITZERLAND

Carol Warner
Biochemistry Department
Gilman Hall
Iowa State University
Ames, Iowa 50011

Richard L. Willham
Animal Science
239 Kildee Hall
Iowa State University
Ames, Iowa 50011

Phletus P. Williams
National Animal Disease Center
USDA, ARS
P.O. Box 70
Ames, Iowa 50010

Cheryl A. Winkler
PRI, FCRF/NCI
Room 11-85, Building 500, NCI/FCRF
Frederick, MD 21701

Steve Woskow
Food Technology
210 Dairy Industry
Iowa State University
Ames, Iowa 50011

Ming-Che Wu
University of Illinois
1207 West Gregory Drive
Urbana, IL 61801

William W. Wunder
Department of Animal Science
123 Kildee Hall
Iowa State University
Ames, Iowa 50011

Anlong Xu
Animal Sciences
114 ASL
1207 West Gregory Drive
Urbana, IL 61801

Yuanxin Xu
Biochemistry Department
Gilman Hall
Iowa State University
Ames, Iowa 50011

Betty M. Young
Department of Animal Science
201 Kildee Hall
Iowa State University
Ames, Iowa 50011

Naoya Yuhki
National Cancer Institute
Building 500, Room 11-85
Frederick, MD 21701-1013

Hua James Zhou
Genetics Student
710 Pammel Court
Ames, Iowa 50010

Xiaoling Zhu
Immunobiology
VMRI
Iowa State University
Ames, Iowa 50011

Dean Zimmerman
Animal Science
337 Kildee Hall
Iowa State University
Ames, Iowa 50011

APPENDIX 2 Financial Support

This conference is the second in a series of Molecular, Cellular, and Developmental Biology (MCDB) Symposia sponsored by Iowa State University. We express our thanks for the help provided by the Departments of Animal Science and Biochemistry and Biophysics, and the MCDB Program. We also gratefully acknowledge financial support from the following sources:

BENEFACTORS ($5,000 TO $9,999)

Iowa State University Biotechnology Program
Iowa State University Graduate College
United States Department of Agriculture

SPONSORS ($2,000 TO $4,999)

Campbell Soup Company
Fisher Scientific
National Animal Disease Center

CONTRIBUTORS (LESS THAN $2,000)

American Breeders Service
American Guernsey Cattle Club
American Jersey Cattle Club
Applied Biosystems, Inc.
Arbor Acres Farm, Inc.
Cargill World Wide Poultry (Shaver Poultry
    Breeding Farms, Ltd)
Carl S. Akey Feeds, Inc.
Cetus Corporation
Cobb-Vantress, Inc.
Lilly Research Laboratories (Eli Lilly and Co.)
Farmers Hybrid Co.
H & N, Inc.
Hy-Line Indian River Company
International Minerals & Chemicals Corporation
Land O'Lakes, Inc.
National Pork Producers Council
National Swine Improvement Federation
Nicholas Turkey Breeding Farms
Norden Laboratories
Peterson Farms, Inc.
Pig Improvement Company
Poultry Breeders of America